TRANSACTIONS

—OF THE—

MICHIGAN DENTAL SOCIETY.

TWENTY-SEVENTH ANNUAL SESSION,

—HELD IN—

DETROIT, MARCH 29TH, 30TH & 31ST, 1882.

PUBLISHED BY ORDER OF THE SOCIETY.

F. S. ACKERMAN & CO.,
MICHIGAN DENTAL DEPOT,
29 and 31 State Street,
DETROIT.

H. D. JUSTI'S

SUPERIOR

INSOLUBLE CEMENT.

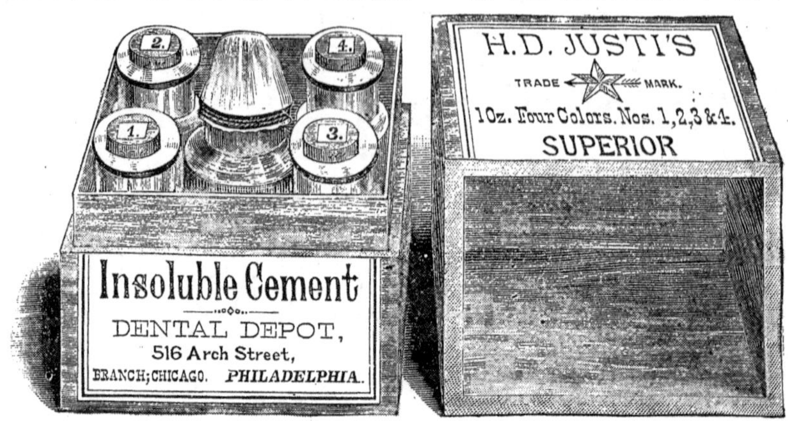

In bringing this **Insoluble Cement** *to the notice of the Dental Profession I do not hesitate to assert, that differing, as it does from all Oxychlorides of Zinc, it is not only equal, but* **Far Superior to any Cement hitherto introduced.**

It becomes harder than any other Cement known, will permanently resist the acids of the mouth, neither expands nor contracts, and attaching itself to the walls of the cavity it prevents the penetration of moisture and arrests decay.

It is composed entirely of non-irritant substances, and exercises a soothing influence, allaying pain when brought in contact with sensitive dentine.

It is made in four different colors, thus enabling the operator to produce any variety of shades, in order to match the patient's tooth.

No. 1—Light. No. 2—Medium. No. 3—Yellow. No. 4—Blue.

PRICES.

1 oz. box,	1 color,	No. 1, 2, 3 or 4,	$3.00
1 " "	4 colors,	" 1, 2, 3 & 4,	3.00
½ " "	1 color,	" 1, 2, 3 or 4,	1.50
½ " "	2 colors,	" 1 & 2 or 3 & 4,	1.50

H. D. JUSTI,
DENTAL DEPOT,

Branch, Chicago, Ill. ***516 Arch St., Philadelphia.***

TRANSACTIONS

—OF THE—

MICHIGAN DENTAL SOCIETY.

TWENTY-SEVENTH ANNUAL SESSION,

—HELD IN—

DETROIT, MARCH 29TH, 30TH & 31ST, 1882.

PUBLISHED BY ORDER OF THE SOCIETY.

F. S. ACKERMAN & CO.,
MICHIGAN DENTAL DEPOT,
29 and 31 State Street,
DETROIT.

DETROIT, MICH.
DETROIT PRINTING COMPANY,
75 Bates Street,
1882.

MICHIGAN DENTAL SOCIETY.

ORGANIZED JANUARY 9th, 1856.

OFFICERS—1882-83.

PRESIDENT—A. T. METCALF,	Kalamazoo.
1st VICE PRESIDENT—W. H. DORRANCE,	Ann Arbor.
2d VICE PRESIDENT—F. W. CLAWSON,	Detroit.
SECRETARY—J. B. McGREGOR,	Port Huron.
TREASURER—J. LATHROP,	Detroit.

COMMITTEES.

EXECUTIVE.

G. R. THOMAS,	Detroit.
E. C. MOORE,	Detroit.
HENRY COWIE,	Detroit.

BOARD OF CENSORS.

G. S. SHATTUCK,	Detroit.
J. A. HARRIS,	Pontiac.
A. M. LONG,	Monroe.

UNIVERSITY VISITING AND CONSULTING COMMITTEE.

J. B. McGREGOR,	Port Huron.
G. L. FIELD,	Detroit.
B. BANNISTER,	Kalamazoo.
E. C. MOORE,	Detroit.
J. A. ROBINSON,	Jackson.

DELEGATES TO THE AMERICAN DENTAL ASSOCIATION.

G. R. THOMAS,	Detroit.
W. H. DORRANCE.	Ann Arbor.
E. C. MOORE,	Detroit.
G. S. SHATTUCK,	Detroit.
J. A. ROBINSON,	Jackson.

MINUTES

OF THE

Michigan Dental Association.

1ST DAY—EVENING SESSION.

DETROIT, MICH., MARCH 29, 1882.

The twenty-seventh annual meeting of the Michigan Dental Association convened in the Russell House parlors at 8 o'clock, P. M., and was called to order by the President, Dr. A. T. Metcalf, of Kalamazoo.

The following candidates were proposed for membership in the Association. Drs. S. C. Case, of Jackson; F. O. Gilbert, Bay City; W. H. Miller, Muskegon and A. W. Eldridge, Big Rapids.

The following members answered to their names at the calling of the roll:

Detroit, Drs. G. L. Field, H. K. Lathrop, Jr., H. Benedict, G. R. Thomas, W. G. Bean, W. C. Britton, H. H. Jackson, J. Lathrop, E. C. Moore, G. S. Shattuck, H. Cowie, J. C. Wood and F. W. Clawson.

Romeo, I. Douglass; Fenton, H. F. Douglass; Ann Arbor, W. H. Dorrance; Jackson, E. Hunter; Adrian, W. H. Knapp and W. Owen; Kalamazoo, A. T. Metcalf; Port Huron, J. B.

McGregor; Grand Rapids, T. R. Perry; Monroe, A. M. Long.

There were also present, as guests of the Association, Drs. Brophy, Talbot, Harlan and Allport, of Chicago; Dr. Barrett, of Buffalo, N. Y.; Dr. Harroun, of Toledo,; Dr. J. Hamilton Thurston, of Jamestown, N. Y., and E. J. Way, of Sandusky, Ohio.

Under the head of Unfinished Business, Dr. E. C. Moore, as Committeeman on Incorporation, read his report. The substance of which was that it was only necessary to file Articles of Association, signed by ten members, and sworn to before a notary public. It was moved by Dr. Thomas, that the report be read and the committee discharged, and report laid on the table; but explained, that he did so for the purpose of bringing the matter before the Association; and offered as his opinion, that it would be for the best interests of the Association to become incorporated, and especially, if we anticipate legislation.

Dr. Talbot, of Chicago, was then introduced to the Association, by the President, Dr. Metcalf. Dr. Talbot having been one of the Committee from the Illinois State Association, in framing a bill, regulating the practice of dentistry in Illinois, and explained to the Association the advantages of the State Association being Incorporated when it came to ask the passage of a law, by the Michigan Legislation in reference to the Practice of Dentistry in this State. Dr. Dorrance and others expressed themselves strongly in favor of incorporation, and for the very reason indicated by Dr. Talbot.

At the request of Dr. Field, Dr. Thomas kindly consented to withdraw (temporarily) his motion, (to receive the report, discharge the committee, and lay the report on the table,) in order that he might make a motion, that the privileges of the floor be extended to visiting members of the profession. Dr. Barrett, of Buffalo, as a visiting member, then explained to the Association the course taken by the New York Dental Association, which was incorporated under a special Act.

He explained further the decided advantage of being incorporated.

Dr. Benedict said that the Michigan Association could get no special legislation, but must become incorporated under the existing State laws. Dr. Moore stated that there would probably be no difficulty in getting a special Act passed by the legislature, under which we could incorporate. The President, Dr. Metcalf, thought that little trouble would be experienced in securing the passage of a special Act, unless special and unusual privileges were asked of the legislature. After some further discussion the report was tabled.

Secretary Moore's and Treasurer Lathrop's annual reports were submitted in a printed form, and were adopted.

There being a vague recollection among some of the older members that the Association was incorporated it was moved by Dr. Hunter, and seconded, that Dr. Field be requested to ascertain whether or not the Association is not already an incorporate body, and report at the session on Thursday. Motion prevailed.

The time had now arrived for the election of officers and selecting the place of the next meeting, but owing to the absence of several members, and a pressure of other important business, it was deemed advisable to postpone this order of business for the present.

Drs. Clawson and Long, were then appointed by the Chair to act as censors for the evening.

The Association then adjourned until 9 o'clock, Thursday morning.

MORNING SESSION.

9 O'CLOCK.

Thursday, March 30th, 2d day.

The Association was called to order by the First Vice-President, Dr. Dorrance.

The Secretary read the minutes of the evening session, which were approved.

The following applications for membership were then read by the President, which took their usual course, and were referred to the Board of Censors:

J. B. DeVries, D.D.S., -	Holland, Mich.
C. F. Porter, " - -	Bay City.
Miss H. L. Martindale, D.D.S.,	Grand Rapids.

Dr. Shattuck, from the Board of Censors, then reported favorable on all the applicants named at this and the evening session, and the following were by ballot elected:

F. O. Gillert, - -	Bay City.
C. S. Case, - - -	Jackson.
W. H. Miller, - -	Muskegon.
A. W. Eldridge, - -	Big Rapids.
B. J. DeVries, - -	Holland.
Harriet L. Martindale, -	Grand Rapids.
C. F. Porter, - -	Bay City.

When Dr. Martindale was declared elected, First Vice-President, Dr. Dorrance, occupying the chair, called attention to the fact that the election of a lady, to membership, is a new experience in the history of the Association, and asking Miss Martindale to arise and be introduced to the Association.

The regular business of the session in order being then taken up, Dr. L. C. Whiting, introduced a few notes with referance to treatment of the six-year molars; the subject was then discussed until the close of the morning session.

The President, *pro tem*, suggested an Obituary Committee on the death of Dr. D. C. Hauxhurst, and by order of the Association appointed the following as members of that Committee:

Dr. I. Douglass,
" G. R. Thomas,
Prof. J. Taft.

The Committee to report at the next session.

The Association then adjourned until 2 o'clock.

AFTERNOON SESSION.

2 O'CLOCK.

Thursday, March 30th, 2d day.

Dr. Dorrance, called the Association to order. The minutes of the morning session were then read by the Secretary, and approved.

The following were proposed for membership of the Association:

W. A. Dumas, - -	Detroit.
F. A. Wilson, D.D.S., -	Grand Rapids.
O. G. Williams, - -	" "
C. R. Rowley, - - -	Niles.

Referred to the Board of Censors.

In the course of the regular order of business, the subject of the First Permanent Molars was taken up and discussed by Drs. Dorrance, Barrett, Taft and others.

Dr. Wilson, of Grand Rapids, then read a paper on the treatment of Deciduous Teeth, which was discussed at length.

At 5 o'clock the discussion was suspended, and Dr. Field's report was received; showing that the Association has been incorporated for a period of 30 years, commencing with the year 1876. The report was accepted and the committee discharged.

The Board of Censors then reported favorably on the following, who were elected:

C. R. Rowley, - -	Niles.
F. A. Wilson, - - -	Grand Rapids.
O. G. Williams, - -	" "
W. A. Dumas, - -	Detroit.

Drs. Barrett, of Buffalo; Brophy, Talbot, Harlan and Allport, of Chicago; Dr. J. A. Moody and Mrs. Dr. K. C. Moody, of Mendota, Ill., were also elected honorary members of the Association.

The Secretary having previously purchased a new book, into which the revised constitution had been copied, it was now suggested that the members sign it, giving the older members the preferance of signing it first.

On motion, the election of officers was made the first order of business on assembling in the evening.

Adjourned to 7:30 o'clock in the evening.

EVENING SESSION.

7:30 O'CLOCK.

Thursday, March 30th, 2d day.

The Association was called to order by the President, A. T. Metcalf.

After the approval of the minutes of previous session, the Secretary read a letter from Mrs. Dr. Stone, of Albion, stating that her husband was ill and unable to attend the meeting of the Association. The letter was ordered filed.

Letters expressing regrets at not being able to be present from Drs. Rehwinkel, Chillicothe, O.; Prof. J. Richardson, Terre Haute, Ind.; and Geo. W. Keely, Oxford, O.; M. F. Finley, Washington, D. C.; L. P. Haskell and Geo. H. Cushing, Chicago; Butler and Ambler, Cleveland; H. A. Smith, Cincinnati, O.; C. S. Chittenden, Hamilton, Ont., and many others, among which is the following, which is quite characteristic of him, whom to know is to love:

XENIA, O, March 27th, 1882.

DEAR FRIEND:

The milder weather has done something, but not enough. I can't go. From neck down to toes there is nearly constant toothache, or something equivalent; my head is easy enough to go, but it is fastened on, so I can't send it. If you find a heart, some affections, and several strong inclinations running about loose, count them mine. Indeed, if you find a stray spirit of a rather friendly cast lingering near, like Mary's little lamb, treat it kindly for my sake. My dilapidated carcass will not be with you.

May our Father in Heaven bless you all!

Your Brother,

GEO. WATT.

The election of officers being the special order of business of the evening, the Association then proceeded to the election of officers for the ensuing year, with the following result:

A. T. METCALF—PRESIDENT, - -	Kalamazoo.
W. H. DORRANCE—FIRST VICE-PRESIDENT,	Ann Arbor.
F. W. CLAWSON—SECOND VICE-PRESIDENT,	Detroit.
J. B. McGREGOR—SECRETARY, - -	Port Huron.
J. LATHROP—TREASURER, - - -	Detroit.

The next meeting of the Association will be held in Detroit, commencing the evening of the last Wednesday in March.

The term of office of Dr. J. A. Watling, of Ypsilanti, as member of the Board of Censors, having expired, Dr. Long, of Monroe, was elected to fill the vacancy; and Dr. Robinson, was elected to fill the vacancy caused by the expiration of Dr. Shattuck's term of office, as a member of the University Visiting and Consulting Committee.

The President appointed Drs. Dorrance, Robinson and Shattuck, a committee to select delegates to the American Dental Association.

President Metcalf then offered the following:

Resolved, That the thanks of this Association are due to E. C. Moore, for his kindness in performing the office of Secretary during the interval caused by the resignation of Dr. M. F. Finley.

The President was then called away on important committee business, when Dr. Dorrance was again called to the chair.

The consideration of regular topics for discussion being in order, the subject of Deciduous Teeth was further discussed, after which the Association adjourned until 9 o'clock, Friday morning.

MORNING SESSION.

9 O'CLOCK.

Friday, March 31st, 3d day.

The Association was called to order by Dr. Dorrance. The minutes of previous session were read and approved. There being no applications for membership, or report from Board of Censors, the Association proceeded under the head of Miscellaneous Business.

Dr. Clawson, moved that Dr. Harroun be made an active instead of an honorary member. Motion seconded by Dr. Shattuck, and carried.

The Special Committee, appointed by the Chair to draft resolutions on the death of Dr. D. C. Hauxhurst, were not ready to report owing to the absence of one of the committee having the report.

Dr. Benedict, offered a resolution, which was accepted; to increase the University Visiting and Consulting Committee, to five members, instead of three, two of said committee shall be elected each year.

A communication was then received from F. S. Ackerman & Co., offering to publish the transactions of the Association, for this year, free of charge to the Association. The communication received, and offer accepted.

The Association then proceeded to ballot for additional committeemen on the University Visiting and Consulting Committee, resulting in favor of E. C. Moore and B. Bannister.

Dr. McGregor then read a paper on "The Relation of Dentistry to Medicine," which elicited a long discussion.

Drs. Allport, of Chicago, and Edson and Evans, Toledo, then arrived.

Dr. Taft moved, that the discussion of the subject of Dr. McGregor's paper be continued until 12:30, and at that time be permanently passed. Carried.

Adjourned at 12:30 to 2 o'clock, P. M.

AFTERNOON SESSION.

2 O'CLOCK.

Friday, March 31st, 3d day.

The minutes of the morning session were read and approved. The Special Committee to draft resolutions of respect to the memory of Dr. Hauxhurst not yet being ready to report, were censured by the Chair, for their apparent neglect in this particular.

Dr. Taft then constituted himself a committee of *that* committee, to hunt up the committeeman having the report in his hands.

As contemplated in the morning session, the subject of "Artificial Crowns on Natural Roots," was then taken up, and Second Vice-President Clawson, was called to the Chair while Dr. Dorrance made some remarks on the above topic, and illustrated them on the black-board in colored crayon. Dr. Talbot, of Chicago, then made some remarks and illustrated on the black-board his peculiar way of mounting crowns; he also gave the names of the originators of the process of mounting crowns.

The Association then took a recess until 7 o'clock, the time agreed upon for the reading of the "History of Dentistry in Michigan," by the historian, Dr. A. T. Metcalf.

EVENING SESSION.

7 O'CLOCK.

Friday, March 31st, 3d day.

The Association was called to order by the President, Dr. Metcalf. The minutes of the previous session were read and approved.

The Special Committee to draft resolutions on the death of Dr. Hauxhurst then made their report as follows:

WHEREAS: Intelligence has come to us that Dr. D. C. Hauxhurst died in Paris, France, February 16th, 1882. Therefore,

Resolved: That in as much as it has seemed good to Him who doeth all things well, that our friend and brother dentist should thus early be removed by death; therefore,

Resolved: That by his death we have lost a fellow laborer in dentistry, of rare attainments for one of his years, whose whole soul was devoted to his profession. Possessing as he did, an amiable, courteous and generous disposition, he was only known to be loved by all. We shall ever fondly cherish his memory, and greatly deplore his loss.

Resolved further: That the sympathies of this Association be extended to his bereaved wife, and aged mother who, will ever honor his memory.

Resolved, That a copy of these resolutions be presented to the above mentioned afflicted ones.

ISAAC DOUGLASS,
J. TAFT,
G. R. THOMAS,
Committee.

The Treasurer's report was then read and accepted, and the following Committees were then appointed by the President:

PUBLISHING COEMITTEE.

F. W. Clawson,
Geo. L. Field,
C. S. Case.

EXECUTIVE COMMITTEE.

G. R. Thomas,
E. C. Moore,
Henry Cowie.

After the appointment of the above Committees, the President then proceeded to read his historical report, which occupied about an hour and a halfs time, but was very interesting, particularly to the older members of the Association. At the conclusion of the reading of the historian's sketch, Dr. Clawson (in the absence of the First Vice President) was called to the Chair: when it was moved, seconded and carried by a two-thirds vote that Dr. Metcalf's resolution of the year previous, regarding the abolition of the Chair of Mechanical Dentistry in the University of Michigan, be taken from the table. Immediately following this, Dr. Metcalf offered as a substitute for his resolution of the year previous, the following:

WHEREAS: that part of our practice known as Mechanical Dentistry, when so constructed as to give the patients the highest attainable results, has become so intricate and complicated, that it cannot be properly learned in the time now devoted to the teaching of it in our Dental Colleges. And,

WHEREAS: in consequence of the insufficient instructions now given, it tends to cheapen, belittle and degrade it. Therefore,

Resolved: that the Officers of this Association and the visitors to the Dental Department of the University of Michigan, are hereby instructed to make all proper efforts to have Mechanical Dentistry taught as a distinct calling, and when students have become proficient in its various departments, that they be entitled to receive a certificate to practice it, regardless of their qualifications to practice Dental Surgery.

At the concluding of the reading of his resolution, Dr. Metcalf was asked to make some remarks in support of his resolution, it being so at variance with the former resolution which had slumbered so unpeacefully for a year on the table; but the time having arrived for the banquet which was now ready, the President availed himself of his official position and suggested that a motion to adjourn was in order, which was offered, seconded and carried, thereby diplomatically nipped in the bud (what might have been) some very flowery speeches.

The Association then headed by the Charter members, adjourned to the banquet room, where an elegant spread awaited them, and after a blessing by Dr. Taft, partook of an elegant supper.

The Toast Master, Dr. Thomas, then commenced assigning toasts, which were responded to in a manner that would do credit to a school of Grecian Orators.

TOASTS AND SENTIMENTS.

The City of Detroit:—

May her beauty ever be equalled by her prosperity.

DR. WM. CAHOON,
Detroit.

The Press:—

The safe guard of liberty and the vehicle of knowledge.

F. J. IRLAND,
Detroit Post & Tribune, City Editor.

The Pioneers of Dentistry:—

" Smile at their first small ventures as we will.
The school-boy's copy shapes the scholar's hand.
Their grateful memory fills our hearts to-day."

DR. C. B. PORTER,
Bay City.

The relation that medicine bears to dentistry:—

" All are but parts of one stupendous whole."

DR. W. W. ALLPORT,
Chicago,

Dental Literature :—

" Diffusiveness without concentration should be avoided. Words may be fluently used without conveying ideas."

DR. W. C. BARRETT, Buffalo, and
DR. EUGENE S. TALBOT, Chicago

Dental Education :—

" A *little* learning is a dangerous thing,
Drink deep, or touch not the Piærian spring."

DR. J. LATHROP,
Detroit.

Dental Students :—

" In the long run fame finds deserving man,
The lucky wight may prosper for a day,
But in good time merit leads the van,
And vain pretence unnoticed goes its way,
There is no Chance, no Destiny, no Fate,
But Fortune smiles on those who work and wait,
In the long run."

PROF. W. H. DORRANCE,
Ann Arbor.

The Past, Present and Future of the Dental Profession :—

" For the structure that we raise,
Time is with materials filled,
Our to-days and yesterdays,
Are the blocks with which we build."
" Build *to-day* then, strong and sure
With a firm and ample base;
And ascending and secure
Shall to-morrow find its place."

DR. J. A. ROBINSON,
Jackson.

Dental Colleges :—

" May their advance be steady.
Unhindered by retreat."

PROF. J. A. WATLING.

The Dentist's leisure hours :—

" Man never *is*, but always *to be* blest."

DR. H. COWIE,
Detroit.

The relation and influence of the older practitioners to the younger:—

"Thou shalt rise up before the hoary head, and honor the face of the old man."

DR. TRUMAN W. BROPHY,
Chicago.

Dental Ethics and Etiquette:—

"Let no mean jealousies pervert your mind,
A blemish in another's fame to find,
Be grateful for the gifts that you possess,
Nor deem a rival's merits makes yours less."

DR. GEO. L. FIELD,
Detroit.

Dental Legislation:—

"The mills of the Gods grind slowly.
But they grind exceeding small,
Though with patience He stands waiting,
With exactness grinds he all."

PROF. J. TAFT,
Cincinnati, O.

Dental Societies:—

"In Union there is strength."

DR. C. H. HARROUN,
Toledo, O.

Mechanical Dentistry:—

"Whose end both at the first, and now, is to hold as 'twere, the mirror up to nature."

DR. E. C. MOORE,
Detroit.

Our duty to our patients:—

"Let patience have her perfect work."
"Words fitly spoken are like apples of gold."

DR. J. HAMILTON THURSTON,
Jamestown, N. Y.

Dental Hygiene in the Public schools:—

"Precept must be upon precept,
Precept upon precept,
Line upon line, line upon line,
Here a little, and there a little."

PROF. W. N. HAILMANN,
Detroit

Among those present from abroad were the following well known dentists: Drs. Allport, Brophy, Talbot and Harlan, from Chicago; Barrett, of Buffalo; Wayc, of Sandusky, O.; Thurston, of Jamestown, N. Y.; Edson and Evans, of Toledo; Prof. Taft, of Cincinnati; Douglass, of Wisconsin, and "Tim Tooley" alias Lenox, of Chatham, Ont.

PAPERS AND DISCUSSIONS

OF THE

Michigan Dental Association

TREATMENT OF SIXTH YEAR MOLARS.

BY DR. WHITING.

I have a few suggestions to present on this subject that may perhaps be of interest to the members of the Association. Something more than the present preservation of these teeth must be looked after, if the future generations are to have teeth at all. These teeth are failing because there is no demand for them in the mastication of our food. As a rule if the parents have good teeth the children will inherit them, but they must be used if they are to be kept in a healthy condition. Nature soon ceases to supply where there is no demand. We have in all our best cities schools, for the development of our physical systems. We must invent some gymnastics for the teeth, or we shall soon have a race of men who have none. To know how to treat these teeth we must know the cause of their decay. I wish to call your attention to one of the most active elements in their destruction, and that is glucose or grape sugar: this is used to adulterate all our candies, syrups and low grades of sugar, and is largely sold by our grocers as "corn goods." This is a branch of the subject which I hope to hear well discussed.

DR. PERRY—Will the Doctor be kind enough to explain how grape sugar has a tendency to increase the decay of the teeth?

DR. WHITING—Grape sugar is manufactured from starch, and the material used in converting starch into glucose is sulphuric acid. In the process this sulpuric acid is not all taken out, a large percentage remains, and sulphuric acid is an active property in the destruction of the teeth.

DR. CLAWSON—The subject we are discussing is the treatment of sixth year molars. I do not see that they require any special treatment any more than other teeth, though of course, they erupt at a time when all the bony structure is soft; but the same rule which wė observ in saving othere teeth, ought to apply to sixth year molars. Dr. Whiting speaks of sulphuric acid in the glucose, my impression is that sulphuric acid is not as injurious as some of the other acids in causing decay. I am quite partial towards sulphuric acid and find it is of use many time, especially in calculi.

DR. SHATTUCK—Dr. Whiting seems to rely on the acid theory of decay entirely. We should remember that decay is a vital as well as a chemical action, that we have to look at the system of our patients, as well as the substances which come in contact with the teeth. As far as sulphuric acid is concerned, we are taught that white decay or light decay, as it is called, comes from nitric acid, while dark decay comes from sulphuric acid. We all know that dark decay is much slower in its ravages, and that these sixth year molars generally decay with the light decay, and I do not know whether it would be proper to charge it to the action of sulphuric acid or not.

DR. BARRETT—Mr. President and Gentlemen: The general subject of the treatment of sixth year molars and their preservation or their sacrifice, has been a vexed question in dentistry for some time. I know that qualified practitioners, men who are ordinarily conservative in their treatment of other teeth, sometimes advocate the extraction of sixth year molars as a rule, whether decayed or not. Their argument is this, that these teeth are apt to be attacked by caries and that their salvation is rather problematical; that by their early sacrifice the neighboring teeth may be brought into line and become serviceable, when otherwise there would be an undue crowding It has always seemed to me, that that line of reasoning was very fallacious. I have always thought, that in the development of the human species there were not too many teeth; that the great prototype, the highest type of development is more than thirty-two teeth, that it is forty-eight teeth, with more permanent molars. In men, however, we have but thirty-two teeth, and the sixth year molar occupies the most important position in the mastication of the food. It is immediately opposite the mouth of the great duct, which supplies the principal portion of the saliva for the preparation of the food, and we all know, that saliva has a most important part to perform in the office of digestion. It is not simply that it prepares the food for deglutition. It is not that it keeps the mouth in a moist condition. It plays a most important part in changing the starch of food to sugar. This tooth, the sixth year molar, is directly opposite the mouth of Steno's duct; therefore it is the most important tooth in that point of view, as in mastication, the food is more freely mixed with the saliva which exudes and is therefore in a more proper condition for digestion. Then it is the largest tooth in the center of the arch, and when that tooth is gone, the principal one in the whole wall has been removed, although if it be taken out sufficiently early, the second molar will come forward and in a great measure take its place. Yet it almost universally stands at an angle. Consequently, I think the sixth year molar should be retained, and such practitioners as recommend its removal are in error, at least from my standpoint.

With reference to decay, I think the idea is becoming more and more prevalent that it is nothing more or less than chemical solution and disintegration. There are other things of course which hasten or hinder it. An hereditary diathesis has its influence. Yet the main principle involved is a chemical principle, and the decay of the teeth is mainly a solution of the lime salts through the action of such acids as are formed in the mouth. As to sulphuric acid, and the Doctor's criticism upon that, has touched me on a tender point. Buffalo is the center and initial point of the glucose manufacture. I have been all through these manufacturies; and I have examined the process and I have examined it as thoroughly and critically as it was in my power to do. Every facility has been placed at my disposal. I made all the tests that I desired to make. This making of glucose is one of the simplest things in the world. We all know that starch, as starch, cannot be digested. Some of my friends know that I have been considerably interested in vivisections, and I have made a good many experiments in that direction, and it is the universal rule that when starch in solution is injected into the system of any of the inferior animals, it always appears as starch. The iodine test for starch always shows it, consequently it is not digested as starch. In the process of digestion it is converted into grape sugar, which is glucose, nothing more or less; and in the manufacture of glucose the process by which it is made is simply the conversion of the grain into starch, then the process of fermentation is begun, but arrested at a peculiar point, the starch is then put into a converter and is treated with sulphuric acid. It is not necessary to go through the whole process, but after the conversion of the starch, and as one of the essential processes, the sulphuric acid is neutralized by carbonate of lime which is put in, in excess, and any acid which may be left is, of course, converted into sulphate of lime, which is insoluble. So I hold glucose to be one of the most harmless, one of the most nutritive, one of the best foods that we have, and its discovery, the discovery of the process of making it, is a thing which should rank among the great discoveries of the world. It gives us an artificial food which we did not have before. It is in a very nutritive and easily digestible form, more digestible than plain sugar. Chemically there is no difference between grape sugar and cane sugar. The former is just as nutritive and more easily digested than the latter, and I believe that if more of our candy was made from grape sugar, instead of cane sugar, it would be better for those who eat it. I know there is a prejudice upon the part of many that too much candy is injurious; giving too much taffy either to children or grown people is considered injurious, and I am not at all sure but that is the case, still it is not the grape sugar that does the harm or any sugar; but it is the leaving of it in the mouth and between the teeth which does the mischief. Where there is a want of cleanliness in the teeth the process of fermentation early sets in. There should be no sulphuric acid in the mouth even, although some traces be left in the glucose it will be neutralized by the carbonic acid in the breath, so you have carbonate of lime again. I do not believe that sugar would do any harm if removed from the mouth, but as I say, if either glucose or cane sugar be left between the teeth for any length of time, the process of fermentation sets in, and the result in most cases will be the formation of acetic acid, which I consider one of the most injurious substances in its action upon the teeth. You will also get malic acid, but especially acetic acid. If any of you have experimented by investing teeth in acetic acid more or less dilute, you will see precisely the same effect that you find in ordinary white decay, as it is called; the same removal of the lime salts from the teeth, leaving nothing but the organic material. The inorganic material has been disolved out by these inchoate acids that are there. We cannot always tell by the fact that the mouth may present an alkaline reaction although these acids may have been present and done their destructive work, they may be neutralized by their action upon the lime salts of the teeth, and so the mouth presents a neutral or alkaline reaction when in reality the destructive action of the acids may have taken place.

I hold that in such cases as this, whether it be the sixth year molars, or the others, the great bugbear which we have to fight, the great enemy which stands in our way like a lurking lion of which we are all afraid, and which overcomes the best of us at times, is this acid which is formed in the mouth, from molecular changes induced by fermentation. The sixth year molars are particularly liable to attacks of this kind for a number of reasons. In the first place any one who knows about their development knows that they are developed at a time when the processes of nature are comparatively weak. In the second place the child's teeth are not cleaned as they should be. This is the dentist's great difficutly in regard to children. It is almost impossible to get them to follow directions in this regard, consequently these acids are formed in the mouth. Then from the very fact, as I said, of the defferentiation which goes on in the production of sixth year molars at a weak period, a weak state in the developement of the child, the teeth themselves are apt to be imperfect, and there are little pits in the center of them. The crystals of enamel which cover their surface, which shoot out like little crystals of ice on the surface of freezing water from every point of vantage, do not coalesce perfectly, consequently there are little fissures, little pits which are sufficient to retain enough food to induce the process of fermentation and the formation of an acid which gets in and cuts out the inorganic portions of the teeth, leaving the organic portions to be destroyed by further process of fermentation. So my great apprehension about the decay of teeth is what I have stated. I object most decidedly to the removal of the sixth year molars as a rule. My reason for it is this. The influence of heredity upon the human system from generation to generation is such, that the constant removal of these teeth induces a contraction of the jaw, which goes on increasing from one generation to another, until, if it proceeds long enough, we will have exactly the same trouble with the second molar, the twelfth year molar, and finally some bad dentist will advocate the removal of the twelfth year molar, the sixth year molar, having by that time become altogether rudimentary. The process may be continued until by and by we will have a race of people with no teeth in the mouth at all, though I do not expect we shall live to see that day. The tendency however is in a wrong direction.

Dr. WHITING—There is one thing I wish to say in regard to the Buffalo Glucose Manufacture. You cannot find a pound of glucose in Detroit as glucose; yet you cannot find a gallon of syrup or anything of that kind in the city that is not adulterated with glucose. You cannot find a grade of our cheap sugars which are not adulterated with glucose.

Dr. BARRETT—I object to the word adulteration used in this connection. Dr Whiting is quite right in bringing out discussion of this matter. I would not give a cent for the announcement of axioms or the laying down of principals which no man can dispute. It is only by discussion that we can get new ideas. And the use of the word adulteration implies a lowering of the standard of the materials composing the thing which is adulterated. It carries the idea of making it worse than it would have been if the admixture had not been made. In this case I think the sugar is better for being mixed with the glucose. It is more easily digested, and from a physiological standpoint it is improved. I think it is one of the most harmless and useful foods we have, consequently I believe that cane sugar is better for being mixed with it. Of course the flavor is not the same, and more of it must necessarily be used to produce the same effect that would be produced by pure cane sugar. A larger quantity has to be eaten in order to get the same amount of sweet.

DR. DOUGLASS—I understand that in the making of candies acids are used to prevent the sugar from graining, and that while the acid may be covered up it is not neutralized. I think acetic acid is used and it must remain in the sugar, although its taste is covered up; just as the sour remains when we use sugar to cover up the taste of the sour.

DR. BARRETT—I so understand, but I do not know.

DR. BROPHY—I am very much of the opinion that my friend Dr. Barrett is in error in regard to the acid formed by the decomposition of glucose or grape sugar. In the first place the starch, by the action of ptyaline, is converted into grape sugar or glucose, and then immediately broken up. The chemical formula of starch is C_6, H_{10}, O_5. This is converted into glucose, and with the addition of the equivalents of water, H_2 O it will then be C_6, H_{12}, O_6. That divided by two we have exactly two molecules of lactic acid, or 2 C_3, H_6, O_3. Lactic acid, in my opinion, is a very powerful agent in the disintegration of the teeth by acting on them, being neutralized and thus producing a neutral solution in the mouth. The formula for acetic acid is C_2, H_3, O_2. It is lactic acid and not acetic acid, in my opinion that does the mischief. Where we find to such an extent the disintregation about the margin of the gums, it is caused by the disorganization of the calcium salts in the teeth. About the margin of the sixth year molars, this disintegration more than in almost any other teeth, takes place. I hope this subject will be discussed. I think Dr. Barrett is in error though, in ascribing this disintegration to acetic acid alone.

Dr. Barrett—I did not mean to be so understood that it was acetic acid alone. I only used acetic acid by way of illustration. I said there were other acids, and I think I named malic acid. I do not know whether I named lactic acid or not.

Dr. Brophy—I understood the doctor to say the starch was broken up into acetic acid.

I think this subject of the preservation of the first molars is a very important one indeed. But there are cases in which it is impossible to do so. The great trouble in all these cases is in the lack of proper advice to parents, who largely believe that the sixth year molars are temporary teeth. It is owing to the improper instruction and lack of knowledge. When we get so that we can advise patients and have our advice followed in the same way that physicians do, when we can impress upon parents the importance of attention to the teeth, to the necessity for their care, then we will be able to do far more in the preservation of these very important teeth.

DR. DORRANCE—(In the Chair). The subject under consideration is the treatment of sixth year molars. This is an important subject, and I hope that it will be further discussed.

DR. TALBOT—I would like to say just one word in regard to the use of acid in candies. I think Dr. Douglass asked for information in regard to that subject. Manufacturers as a rule, are not in the habit of using materials for the manufacture of their products which would be detrimental to their own interests. In other words, they are not in the habit of using materials which would decrease their financial prosperity. In regard to the manufacture of candies from glucose this rule holds good. The impression has gone out that sulphuric acid enters largely into the formation of candies, from the fact that it is used, as Dr. Barrett has said in the manufacture of glucose. In the manufacture of candies copper vessels are used. If glucose contains sulphuric acid it would be impossible to use it in these vessels, because it would destroy them. They are very expensive, and manufacturers could not afford to frequently replace them. Therefore I think it is absurd for anybody to suppose that sulphuric acid would be used in the manufacture of candy.

DR. PERRY—While the sixth year molars are of such great importance it is almost impossible always to save them. Then the next best thing is to do the best you can. The thing we most wish to know is how best to preserve them. We are all anxious to learn that. While I do not pretend to be able to permanently save the sixth year molars, I do try to save them as long as possible, at least until the second molars are able to do good service. The one great important thing is to instruct your patient. Circumstances alter cases. While you may be able to preserve the sixth year molars in many cases, there are many of these little ones who come to us, who have not vitality enough to make it possible to preserve them. The teeth do not get nutrition enough. The question then is what shall we do? My practice has been to preserve them as long as possible. I do not think it best, however, to sacrifice the bicuspids and second molars in a futile attempt to save the sixth year old molars. My rule is to preserve the most teeth possible. I always endeavor to preserve these molars until at least the twelfth year. I do not say that the result will always be favorable, and, as my friend Dr. Barrett says, when they are extracted early their neighbors are almost invariably at an angle. This is not always true however. I have had some very fine results by extracting sixth year molars when I saw it was impossible to preserve them after the twelfth year molars had been erupted. As I said the important thing is to preserve the most teeth. I do not say that we can save all, or that the sixth year molar is the most important in the entire mouth; it is a very important tooth, particularly for the first few years. Dr. Barrett has given us a very good idea of what ought to be done in regard to these teeth, and I think those practitioners who extract them in anticipation of decay are in very great error. It is also a great error to endeavor to save all the sixth year molars at the expense of some of the others.

Dr. Douglass—On one point I differ from Dr. Perry. I think if we cannot save the sixth year molars later than the twelfth year, if they are taken out early, the twelfth year molars will almost always take the same position that the sixth year molar occupies, or very nearly so.

Dr. Perry—My experience is that it would invariably have an angle, and the result would be a very small grinding surface; whereas if the extraction is deferred until the twelfth year, the chances are you will have a larger grinding surface.

Dr. Way—So far as I heard, it would seem to be the unanimous opinion that wherever able to do so, we should save the first molars. That is not the opinion of every dentist. We have men in the profession who are supposed to understand these things very well, men whom we look up to who say, that as a rule, the loss of the sixth year molar is inevitable, that it must be lost; that it is therefore better, this being the case, to extract this molar at a certain age, because then the next molar as it is erupted, will largely take its place, will stand perpendicular and present a very much larger surface for mastication. The general idea, so far as we have heard it here, is that it is always best to save the first molar if possible. That is also my opinion. As Dr. Barrett has said, it occupies the most important position in the jaw, and if it can be saved it should remain there. Nature is wiser I presume than any dentist, therefore, if it is best to save that tooth it should be done. But whenever it cannot be permanently saved it is useless to attempt to do it. When it has got beyond salvation there is no use talking, it must go and that is the end of it. The question is, can we take such measures that we may save it? I am of the opinion that in more cases than we think, it is possible to save it, but that depends upon the care the teeth receive at an early age. I think if parents can be taught to take care of their children's teeth from the first, it will greatly simplify our work. Of course, we cannot expect that under the present state of things, the work will be very well done.

Speaking of another branch of this subject it is also important to save the deciduous teeth. There is a reason for that which everyone does not think of. It is very important that these teeth should be saved with the pulps alive until the permanent ones are erupted. The reason is, that the roots of these teeth do not absorb after the nerve is destroyed. The permanent teeth, when they come in, are apt to be deflected to one side or the other, not being erupted as they should be. Of course, we have constitutions so weak that when the sixth year molars are erupted, the material of the teeth seems to be of so inferior a character that they are hardly enabled to resist even the slightest tendency toward decay. The enamel seems scarcely thicker than paper, and is soft and of little use. The grand question, it seems to me, is what shall we do with that class of teeth? These are the teeth we would like most to save, but these are the teeth that are most difficult to preserve. Upon that point I would be happy to obtain information. I wish to put myself on record as being strongly in favor of preserving the sixth year molar under all circumstances when it can be saved.

Dr. Clawson—I beg to differ with the gentleman from Sandusky, in regard to the absorption of the roots of deciduous teeth. I am very well satisfied that they do absorb even after the death of the pulp; that the membrane which surrounds the root will act in this case the same as the pulp would in teeth where the nerve remains. I am quite positive that it is so. I have seen cases where the pulp had been destroyed for some time, and yet it seemed to me that the roots did absorb naturally. I would like to ask the gentleman from Sandusky, speaking about saving deciduous teeth, what his mode of treatment is, and what material he would recommend for filling them. I wish to know if he has made that a specialty?

Dr. Waye.—My opinion is that the main thing is to keep the nerve alive. I am strongly of the opinion, from my own experience, and I am backed by the experience of others in this matter, that absorption of the root ceases upon the death of the nerve.

Dr. Hunter.—In regard to the absorption of the root of a deciduous tooth, after the pulp is dead, I am of the same opinion as Dr. Waye, of Sandusky; and where there is apparent absorption of the root, after the death of the pulp for any length of time, I believe it is not absorption, but necrosis that produces that appearance upon the root. We all know that when that process is perfectly performed there is no such appearance upon the root of the tooth as there is where it has been left in the mouth for a long time after the death of the pulp. It is a vital process, and is perfectly performed.

I am in favor of saving the pulps of deciduous teeth alive. With reference to the saving of the first permanent molar, the course that the discussion has taken has placed us in a terrible dilemma. We claim to be a scientific body. We claim to be working for the benefit of humanity. Yet, right here, on this most important question, with reference to saving the sixth year molar, the opinion is divided, and the discussion is on the balance. Are we working for our pockets, or are we working for humanity? Are we inquiring into the subject from a scientific standpoint? Are we working with reference to benefiting humanity in the future, or simply the patient that comes under our hand? Are we thinking men, or are we mere mechanics and operators, working for the sake of passing the time, and putting money into our pockets? These are questions that come pressing upon us and demand an answer. We must go to the bottom of the subject. We must study it in a scientific way. We must go further back than we have been accustomed to go. We must inquire into pre-natal physiology. We must inquire what functions are performed previous to the birth of the child. We know that the mentality of the race is determined previous to that time. If that is so we have a right to infer that the character of our physical systems is determined previous to that time. If this can be established by facts and by argument, we, as dentists, are under obligation to carry on our investigations upon ground that has been considered sacred.

When we study our science as we should, I believe it will come to this. We must go back further than the time of the eruption of the first permanent molars. We must go back and inquire into the causes. It is a long way, and we cannot go over the whole ground in a short time. This is going to be the labor of the dentists who follow us. we cannot accomplish much in that great work, but we can at least start in that direction.

DR. OWEN.—I would like to put myself on record as believing in the absolute necessity of of saving the six year old molars if practicable. I think a great deal must be done by education. All of us who have practiced dentistry long, know that a great majority of these cases come to us as the first teeth to be cared for. Very few parents pay any attention to the matter until the child has the toothache. When they take the trouble to make an examination they find that the tooth is decayed. They suppose that of course it is one of the temporary teeth, and let it go. We must instruct parents more in the idea of looking after these teeth in early childhood.

I am a very great advocate of saving the deciduous teeth in life until nature designed they should be out, and I think it can be done in a great many instances. The question has been asked as to the kind of filling it is best to use. There are a great many things which are well adapted to the purpose. I have had very good success with phosphate of zinc. I do not use hard fillings, because generally, with children, you cannot do justice to them; but if you can bridge over the difficulty for two or three years, or sometimes for a few months, thus protecting the nerve, you save the vitality of the tooth. If a child loses its teeth when from four to five years of age, it cannot have the proper development of the jaw. The jaw contracts, and before it would get the six year old molar, the contraction would be so great as to leave scarcely room for them, or for the bicuspids. Keep the deciduous teeth as long as possible. That is my theory, and though I do not always practice it I always advocate it. My reason for using phosphate of zinc filling is that it does not irritate so much as some other soft filling.

Dr. Perry.—I see several gentlemen are wishing to be put upon record as to the desirability of saving the six year old molars. I do not think there is any controversy in that respect at all. The question is, how best and longest to preserve them. If they cannot be preserved through life, preserve them as long as possible.

Dr. McGregor.—I would like to ask Dr. Waye, of Sandusky, who believes that no absorption takes place after devitalization of the deciduous teeth, whether he would recommend the removal of those teeth after he found that the vitality was lost, and run his risk of the twelvth year molar forcing its way through into its proper position, or whether he would recommend its removal at once for fear that the molar might be deflected from its course in the way he referred to.

Dr. Waye.—I should be governed altogether by the circumstances. I see no reason for removing a tooth simply because I knew that the pulp was no longer alive, provided it created no irritation or disturbance in any way. It would depend largely upon circumstances. Usually a child needs its teeth for the purposes of mastication, and unless there are some good reasons why it should be removed, a tooth should remain.

Dr. Clawson.—I am satisfied that deciduous teeth are as capable of anti-septic treatment as any others. If such is the case where the pulp has been removed, and yet there is vitality in the surrounding membrane, I see no good reason why deciduous teeth, if properly treated, could not be preserved on the same principle as any others.

Dr. Taft.—I wish to say a few words in reference to the so-called sixth year molars. First, I would say, that the name had better be changed, and the tooth should be known as the first permanent molar. I think that is a far more distinctive name, and one which conveys a more accurate idea. I do not like the expression "six year *old* molar;" why not talk about the "twelve year *old* molar," or the "eighteen year *old* molar." I do not know that you all emphasize the *old*. It seems to me this use of the term should be abandoned, and that we should take up one that is significant, that is sufficiently distinctive at least to convey the idea as to what tooth is meant. If we use the term "first permanent molar," it can be mistaken by no one. I know the other name has been used for a long time, but that is no reason why we should keep on using it, why we should continue it longer.

In regard to these particular teeth, I hardly see the occasion of making them so prominent as has been done, or why the treatment for their preservation should differ from that of others. It is true these teeth come at a time when they are peculiarly liable to the attacks of decay. It is true, perhaps, that the early removal of them, or their removal at an earlier period than some of the other teeth, results in a change of position; but, after all, the removal of any tooth in the mouth at an early time in life, is likely to be followed by a change in the position of its neighbors. It is not the first permanent molar alone whose removal is followed by a change of position in its anterior or posterior neighbor. This very frequently occurs upon the removal of these teeth, and perhaps more frequently than in any other instance, except in cases of teeth erupted at the same period. That the change may be a little more apparent in this case there is no doubt, because of the early period of life at which it comes. Especially if removed prior to the time of the eruption and establishment of the second and third molars in position, this is apt to occur. There is very apt to be a change in the position of the adjoining teeth. But the change that takes place in the second molar, and in the bicuspid teeth will depend very much upon the occlusion of the teeth. They will sometimes remain stubbornly in position entirely unyielding. Sometimes the anterior and posterior teeth will almost wholly occupy this space occasioned by the removal. I have in a great many instances, where teeth were removed at twelve years of age, seen the second molar and the second bicuspid remain stubbornly in position, no closure being made of the space made by the removal of the first molar. In such cases the occlusion is such as to perhaps hold them in position, or they may be so firmly fixed in their sockets that they cannot readily be removed. Then again, some persons make much more use of their teeth than others. These teeth have a greater lateral motion. They move on themselves to a greater extent than in other cases, and these differences of condition cannot fail to have some influence in changing the position of the teeth. I have no doubt either of the fact that in a great many intances the very marked change that occurs in the position of the teeth is due to the fact that the first permanent molars were early removed. About that there is no doubt. As to the utility of preserving them there is no doubt. There are few indeed who would ruthlessly take these teeth away without some very good reason. The propriety of removing them, the circumstances which would render their removal desirable, or important, or necessary, would be about the same as in the case of a bicuspid, or a second molar, or a third molar. It would seem then, that it is hardly necessary to single out this tooth and make it the object of so much discussion, and giving it so much importance over the other teeth, talking about them, in fact, as if they were hardly worth preserving.

It is true, as has been said, that when these teeth come under the care of a dentist they are frequently very much decayed, but that is also true of any tooth in the mouth. Frequently when the second molars come under the care of a dentist they are also very much decayed, and the same is true of the bicuspids, especially of the first bicuspids; perhaps I might say especially of any tooth in the mouth. Perhaps under some circumstances the decay of the first permanent molar is of more frequent occurrence than in any tooth in the mouth. Some statistics bearing upon this subject would seem to indicate this, while other statistics indicate that other teeth in the mouth decay more frequently. There may be various circumstances which will modify these peculiarities of decay, and the teeth which it attacks. Habits of life modify these conditions to some extent. That these teeth decay very frequently there is no doubt. They should be treated much the same as any other teeth in the mouth. They should be kept in the mouth as long as possible. I think the better method, in a majority of cases, would be to protect and preserve these teeth as long as possible for the sake of the neighboring teeth. Occasionally it will occur that when the first molar is removed the second will come squarely up to position. The bicuspid will drop back a little, and the space will be well occupied to a greater or less extent—sometimes wholly occupied. There are all degrees between the complete occupancy and the non-occupancy. The cases in which the other teeth will come squarely up and keep their places are exceptional indeed. The chief difficulty is that while there may be a change of position in the bicuspids and second molar, they are inclined a little and approach each other at an angle. I would prefer ordinarily that there should be no movement of the bicuspid and second molar at all rather than that kind of a movement. It throws the occlusion out of joint, and the ability to masticate with such teeth is very small indeed. It is much impaired at any rate. Unless they come together sufficiently to satisfactorily occupy the entire space, it would be better that these teeth should stand squarely in position and present a true grinding surface. The first molar should be preserved as long as possible, and its removal deferred until it seems an absolute necessity. In a very great many instances, indeed, it is better to preserve even the roots of the first molars, if healthy, and if they can be preserved, for the sake of the neighboring teeth. I know that the practice is strongly urged by many that when the first permanent molar is so much decayed that there is no hope of preserving it, it should be taken out at once. That, it seems to me, is a fallacious theory. Others again, when the first permanent molar is decayed but a little, take it out because of what it will do. No other teeth are so treated. Other teeth have the very best efforts put forth for their preservation, when decay attacks them in its incipiency or is discovered in its more advanced stages of progress. The same rule should be followed with the first molars. All that can be done, all that promises any good results for their preservation should be done, as long as they can be of any service. In a great many instances I feel it is better to preserve even the roots of these teeth to keep them in good position, than ruthlessly to take them out prematurely. To do this I regard as disastrous in almost every instance. There are cases, perhaps, in which there would seem to be strong reason for their removal for a correction of irregularity. But under ordinary circumstances it is better, and the most good is accomplished, to preserve the roots as well as possible rather than to take them away, unless a tooth is very much out of position. I think the removal of the first molar will many a time operate disastrously to the teeth on either side. This of itself is a strong argument for retaining these teeth. It is important that the teeth should be uniform, and where anything occurs to destroy this uniformity—to prevent any tooth from having a corresponding one on the other jaw—it is a misfortune. The removal of these molars oftentimes occasions contraction of the whole jaw, whereas the preservation of the roots, even when the crown may be hardly worth saving, will prevent a disastrous change in the position of the teeth adjoining. Where there is an irregularity in the number of teeth there is a tendency to masticate upon the other side, if it can be done with more ease and greater facility than upon the side where the teeth are absent. Many a time where there is an exposed gum and hard substances strike upon it in the act of mastication, the person will involuntarily avoid using that side of the mouth. I know that experimentally. Due watch should be kept over the teeth to correct any tendency of this kind. Any one who does not give attention to this will soon experience injurious results. On the side of the mouth having the most perfect set of teeth, where there will be the least trouble and irritation, the side that will best perform the work, there is were it will be done. Now, if the roots of these molars can be retained in health, as roots are retained in these advanced days of dental surgery and science, the teeth will be kept in position, and there will be no resulting irritation of the gum, and this tendency to use the teeth upon the opposite side will be largely corrected, even though the whole crown of the tooth does not remain. That is my experience. I have watched that class of teeth quite closely, and I have found it almost universally true that where the root of the first molar remains sound, a person will use the teeth upon that side of the mouth with about the same readiness that the teeth upon the other side are used. For this reason I think it is very important that these roots should be retained. These remarks in reference to the roots of this particular tooth apply with equal force to the roots of any teeth. The facility with which artificial crowns are now applied to the roots of molar teeth draws our attention more especially to the preservation of them.

DR. CLAWSON—I should like to ask Dr. Taft whether he has not sometimes found the roots of these sixth-year molars imperfectly formed, owing to their not being fully developed at an early age, and what he would do in similar cases to that. If, for instance, a nerve had sloughed off; I am much interested to know what he would do in that case, if he did find them imperfectly formed. I have a specimen in my office which illustrates that particular form of case.

DR. TAFT—My advice would be, in such a case, to do the best you can. It is a very easy matter to raise extra or special cases and make special criticism; far more easy to do that than it is to answer them. If you cannot preserve a tooth, let it go, and do the next best thing. Simply endeavor to ascertain what is the best thing to do in all cases, and do that. I know to what you refer—a case where the root has never been completed, and the pulp has become devitalized prior to the development of the harder portion of the root. In cases of this kind the treatment depends very much upon the skill and ability of the individual who has the case to treat. Some men can do things that others cannot do. A good many men can do things that I cannot do—things that I cannot venture upon at all. The question is very frequently asked; Here is a root the pulp of which is dead; the root itself is incomplete. There is a large canal all the way down through to the point of the root. What is to be done in a case of this kind? It is quite likely that if the tooth is filled the root itself will break down. Disease will be produced. The root itself will become decomposed. Just what is the best thing to do in a case of this kind it is hard to say. Unless the opening is entirely too large, the tooth can easily be treated. As I said before, the treatment must depend entirely upon the skill and ability of the operator.

Dr. Douglass—Some of you know that I began my practice of dentistry about thirty years ago in an interior town of the State. I think I have had same advantages that some of you have not had, in consequence of being able to watch my patients for so long a time—some of them. I do not agree with my old friend, Dr. Taft, in one regard, that is in reference to the name these teeth should be called. I know you will not all agree with me, but I think the name sixth-year molars is as appropriate a name as we can have for these teeth. They come about the sixth year of the life of the person. To call them first permanent molars would I think, in most instances, be improper, because they are so temporary in their existence, a large portion of them being lost within a few years, being past redemption when the dentist is first called upon to treat them. This subject is one that was given to me a few weeks ago to prepare a paper upon. My time has been so much occupied that I have been unable to do that. I wish, however, to say a few words upon the subject, and I will now relate a recent case that came under my notice.

A lady came into my office a few weeks ago with her little boy, nine years old. He had lost all the temporary molars but one. He had three bicuspids in the place of the molars that had been lost. The right lower sixth-year molar had been extracted some time previous, in consequence of an abcess having formed at the apex of the roots. The left sixth-year molar was very badly decayed. There was a large crowno-buccal cavity—if I may be allowed the expression—extending below the gums and nearly to the roots. A semi-fungus growth of gum filled almost the entire cavity. The child had been suffering for months very severely from that tooth. I found that if that tooth was removed there were no teeth left that articulated well. The upper central incisors were in place and fully developed in appearance. The upper lateral incisors were neither of them erupted. All of the lower incisors were erupted to their full extent—that is the central ones were. The lateral incisors below were only just erupted about one-third the length of the crown. As I say, if this lower sixth-year molar was lost, he had no two teeth that articulated well. The second bicuspid on the right side of the lower jaw partially articulated with the upper sixth-year molar. The pulp of the tooth, in which the cavity had formed, was in such a highly inflamed condition that the least touch upon the semi-fungus growth of gums that filled the cavity gave very severe pain. I very carefully raised the fungus portion, placed under it a pledget of cotton, saturated with creosote, in which had been dissolved sulphate of morphia until it was nearly as thick as honey. I requested them to call again the next day. They did so. By repeated applications of this remedy I increased the size of the pledget until I could place another one over the one loaded with the morphine and creosote, and succeeded in pressing away that gum until it was absorbed—till there was no longer any semi-fungus growth. I did not stop there, but continued in increasing the quantity of cotton applied to the tooth until I had pressed the gum away below the cavity, and caused it to remain there long enough so that I could fill the cavity with phosphate of zinc. By the time I had got the gums pressed away, the sensitiveness of the pulp had subsided enough so that I carefully prepared the cavity for the filling, with very little pain to the little patient, although he was of an extremely nervous disposition, slender and delicate, and exceedingly sensitive to pain, having been sick a great deal. The first time I did any filling for him he became in such an excited state in a very few minutes that after perspiring freely for a little while he became very feverish, and I did not deem it advisable to at once proceed. I stopped, and tried to attract his attention with one thing and another, finally getting him to look at things under a microscope. The feverish condition went down, and he became as quiet as could be. Then I worked for an hour without the excitement coming back again. I persevered until I had filled all the sixth-year molars. This one that I filled with phosphate of zinc was so very bad I afterward cut away a portion of it and filled it with metallic filling. The tooth is apparently in fine condition, the pulp alive, and the boy able to masticate as well as if the tooth had never decayed. In regard to saving the roots of teeth, I agree with my friend, Professor Taft. I consider it very important indeed to save the roots of teeth after the crowns are gone, if they have not come under my care before. Something like twenty-eight years ago I filled the roots of an upper molar after the crown had gone, and a few years ago there was a case came to me where I had filled an upper cuspid which had been ulcerated for some time, with an abcess at the end of the root, discharging through a fistulous opening twenty-three years before. That caused me to have curiosity to know how the roots of this sixth-year molar that I filled twenty-eight years before had got along. So I wrote the lady, who I think lives in Owasso now, to know what the result had been with her tooth. I received reply saying that five years previous to my writing the roots had been extracted in preparing the jaw for a full set. The filling seemed to be perfect, and the tooth had not caused any uneasiness since it was filled. It did its work equally as well as the other teeth. I think we need not be discouraged in our attempts to save these roots.

Sometimes the root may be decayed so that there is a much larger opening at the apex than there would be otherwise. We usually find that is the case with the palatine root of the upper molars, if any.

I adopt the following course to ascertain the length of the root. I mark the exact length on the shaft of the burr that I use in enlarging the opening at the apex, this being as small a burr as I can use. Then I take the next sized larger burr and marking upon the shaft of that just the length of the root, proceed with it until the burr is very close to the apex, as close as I can come and not go through. I then roll a little pellet of gold, pressing it through a hole in a piece of bone or ivory, having a piece with graded holes, and pressing it through one, then another, then another, till I get just the size of the drill or burr last used. I can depend on this piece going just as far as the burr went, and no further, into the tooth. It is then easy to fill on to that as much gold as I please without any trouble. If the root has an abcess formed at the apex of it, I treat that once, and once only, as a rule, by pumping creosote or carbolic acid through the root, and I usually use creosote. I commenced with it, it has done me good service, and I consider it an old friend, feeling inclined to cling to it. I pump creosote into the root until it begins to discharge through the fistulous opening. Then I proceed with the filling of the root at the same sitting, and complete the work. If the abcess does not close up, I then give silicia or phosphorus, or hepar sulphur, whichever seems best, owing to the general condition of the system. I generally give phosphorus. In case I do not succeed with the use of phosphorus in closing up the fistulous opening, I go on with the other remedies. In nine cases out of ten I do succeed in this way, giving the phosphorus internally. I generally give the second or third dilution, in drop doses. After phosphorus, I have given silicia with good results, and in a few instances I have given hepar sulphur with good results. I seldom give the second remedy. For many years I have proceeded in the way I have spoken of, and have then often placed an artificial crown upon the root, although it is decayed to a mere shell. I have introduced one mode of filling for small cavities in childrens' teeth, which saves the nerves of the little fellows very much, and since I have been so successful with it, I have adopted it many times in filling the teeth of adults. We sometimes find one of the sixth year molars, where the appearance of the grinding surface of the crown is as though it had been once in a waxy state, pierced by a great many little fine holes, little pin holes in the crown. By simply drilling out these places and enlarging the cavity below the surface, in one or two directions very slightly, then by fitting this drill to one of the graded holes in a piece of bone or ivory, as I spoke of, then taking my tin foil, or gold, whichever I decide upon, and making a cylinder of it that will go through one of these holes, gradually pressing it through one, then another a little smaller, and another smaller still, till I get it the size of the drill that I use to prepare the cavity with, I form a plug that will just fit the cavity, except for the slight enlargement in the bottom below the surface. I then dry my cavity and introduce this plug, and pack it into the cavity until it is thoroughly solid. In that way it is not necessary to keep the patient's mouth open to exceed three minutes at a time. I have adopted this plan in a great many instances with grown up people. I consider it as perfect a filling as can be put in a tooth in any way. As for the retaining of the sixth-year molars, I don't think they would have been placed there, with the others so much dependent upon them, if they were not needed; and as has been said, if these teeth are removed the others tilt backward or forward according as they are placed anterior or posterior to the sixth-year molars. When they once begin to tilt that way, the use of them in masticating food tends to increase that condition of things, which is, of course, abnormal, until they sometimes become a source of serious annoyance, the continued lateral pressure upon them causing inflammation, and finally an abcess at the root, the teeth having to be sacrificed in consequence. As regards the cause of the decay of these teeth so frequently and so prematurely, we cannot always control that. If we could control and govern the circumstances from the commencement of the development of these teeth, we would be enabled many times to avoid the unhappy results from decay, and there would not be nearly so many malformed teeth. A physician noticing a case of irregularity or malformation of teeth would say it was a mark of scrofula; but I think, as a rule, we may know that it comes from imperfect development. I have often inquired, and have frequently found that just about the time the grinding surface of the tooth was beginning to calcify, the patient was suffering from the dentition, perhaps, of the first temporary incisors. The child may have been very seriously ill at that time, so much so as to interfere very seriously with the nutrition. The child may be suffering from measles, scarlet fever, diphtheria, or miasmatic influence. Either of these may cause imperfect development of the tooth. I have taken pains in a great many instances to inquire what disease the child suffered from at such a time. In numerous cases I have ascertained, to my perfect satisfaction, what the diseased condition was that caused this imperfect development. Sometimes it has been miasmatic influences, sometimes one fever and sometimes another. Many times I have been satisfied it was from an ordinarily diseased condition operating during the eruption of the temporary teeth.

A MEMBER—Do you find that cutaneous diseases always interrupt nutrition?

DR. DOUGLASS—I don't know that I have in a single instance ascertained that the teeth became imperfectly developed in consequence of any cutaneous disease. I have met a few instances where children were suffering from severe cutaneous diseases, and have wished very much to ascertain what the condition of the teeth developed at that time would be. So far, however, I have not had an opportunity to inquire.

Adjourned to 2 o'clock., P M.

AFTERNOON SESSION.

DR. TAFT—In reference to the nomenclature that has been used in speaking of the first permanent molars, I wish to say that I think it is misleading. A great many persons have the idea that these molars are temporary teeth. In many instances when I have spoken to patients of these teeth as being the first permanent molars, they have said, "I did not suppose these were permanent; I supposed they were temporary teeth." I think if we were more accurate in our expressions it would have an educating influence upon the future.

Dr. Barrett—It seems to me that this term "six-year-old molars, or sixth-year molars," is physiologically absurd and professionally despicable. There are no six-year-old molars, nor sixth-year molars. The age at which they are erupted is so uncertain that certainly it is not sufficient to be depended upon. If they were erupted at the seventh year they might just as well be called seventh-year molars, or seven-year-old molars, and we might continue the comparison indefinitely.

Dr. Dorrance—Laying aside all question on the merits of the case, as to the retention of the first permanent molar or its loss, we must often be called upon to decide about the retention of that important tooth. The loss of these teeth at the age when they are usually lost—a short time after eruption—results in serious injury. It results not only in less grinding surface and support to the other teeth, but also in a contraction of the jaw. The jaw is shortened and robbed of its symmetry, and many of us might be much handsomer men than we are now if we had not lost those teeth a good many years ago. The teeth are not only allowed to crowd themselves around toward the side on which the tooth is lost, but the shortening of the jaw results in a deformity, and in some cases in a considerable deformity. Many parents wish this tooth to be extracted because it is a source of so much pain and loss of sleep, not only to the little patient, but to the parents. You must be able to satisfy them that it is proper and best that these teeth should be retained, and you must be able to treat the tooth to the best advantage, so as to save not only the inorganic portions, but the pulp, too. We cannot afford to lose the pulp. This question is a very serious one, because oftentimes the tooth is so frail, not being fully developed, and the conditions are so unfavorable that the operation is a difficult one. Then, too, the patient will not let you do anything without particular urging and coaxing.

DR. HUNTER—I think the only question to be decided in a general treatment of these teeth is whether they were intended to be there; whether they were put into the mouth by infinite wisdom. If so, they should remain there as long as it is possible to retain them by the exercise of all our skill.

DR. TAFT—It is supposed that these teeth are differently situated as regards liability to decay, and as regards their position in reference to the other teeth from any of the others. It seems to me that is the only apology for singling them out and making them the object of distinctive consideration. There are, it is true, some circumstances which attend these teeth which do not attach to the others with perhaps the exception to the anterior teeth, that come at about the same period, and under about the same conditions and embarrassments. The incisors, for example, come at about the same period as the first permanent molars. They are many times subject to the same structural peculiarities. They have the disadvantage of the presence of the temporary teeth, which under certain circumstances is an unfavorable condition. They are erupted at a time when the developing power is not so strong, and when there is more liability to disturbance of nutrition—when the mouth, perhaps, undergoes a disturbance from irritation more than at subsequent periods. These teeth remain for some time in the mouth without special attention on the part of the possessor, while at a later period more care will be given to the teeth which are then in the mouth.

Oftentimes the temporary teeth are decayed, and foreign substances are retained in contact with the permanent molar. Decomposition takes place, and decay producing agents are formed. Again, many times during childhood there may be vitiation of the secretion of the mouth, which is less liable to occur in after years. The first permanent molar will usually have more structural defects than teeth which come later. Frequently the enamel is imperfectly fused. Imperfect tracts are frequently found on the surface. The second and third permanent molars are usually more perfect structurally than the first. These are some of the peculiar circumstances which attach to the first molars, but this can be no sufficient warrant for neglecting them or ruthlessly letting them go. When we have a difficulty to meet, an embarrassment to contend with, we should summon the greater energy to meet the emergency. The success which we will have with these uncetain subjects—the first permanent molars—will often be greater than we can anticipate. In many cases it will be found that our expectations are far exceeded. I remember a case in which I filled the first permanent molar twenty-eight years ago, and it has remained in apparently perfect condition until the present time. I have seen a number of cases of this kind, although, perhaps. not enough of them to predicate a principle upon. It is almost equally true that many times our hopes of ultimate success and permanency will be disappointed. We must understand the underlying principles and be governed by them, rather than any particular cases that may come under our professional care.

I do think that while these teeth are very important, they are not so much more so than others as to justify any very long discussion on the methods of their special preservation. Next year we might take up the treatment of superior central incisors, or lateral incisors, or cuspids. This would be just as consistent, except, indeed, for the fact of these embarrassments I have spoken of that do attach to the first permanent molars.

TREATMENT OF THE DECIDUOUS TEETH.

DR. F. D. WILSON.

The first and greatest difficulty we encounter, perhaps, is in securing the little patient upon which to practice the skill we may possess. Often the first appearance of the infant (?) in the office of the dental practitioner is for the purpose of leaving with him a carious temporary molar, as they think, but which proves to be one of the first members of the permanent set. The dentist who is the possessor of a number of children may consider himself favored in regard to this matter, at least for the experienoe it affords him.

Parents should be instructed to have their children's teeth examined at intervals, from the period that they first begin to erupt.

A mere mention to them is not sufficient. Impress its importance upon their minds.

Mothers have a tenderness for their offspring, for which reason it is easy to find an excuse for neglect.

When a child is taken to a dentist, or he is called upon to visit it, he should first inspire it with confidence in himself. He should be kind, considerate, but firm. He should have a strict regard for the *truth*, and in *no* particular deceive a child.

It should not only be discouraged, but absolutely forbidden for the parent to do so. Tell the child what you intend to do, as near as possible, that it may be painful, and encourage it to bear it. To lose its confidence in you is as bad as to lose the patient.

Let us now examine the jaws of a fœtus. The process of formation of the teeth previous to the deposition of lime is divided into three stages. From six to ten weeks is the papillary stage; from ten to fourteen the follicular; and from fourteen to fifteen the saccular. From the sixteenth to the twenty-first weeks the deposit of lime begins. The teeth are first gradually formed in soft tissues, the crowns becoming calcified before the roots are entirely formed in soft tissue. At birth the two superior maxillar are united by a fibro cartilage.

At the period of the eruption of the first teeth, the crowns of the central incisors are perfected, and the lateral incisors are almost equally advanced. The crowns of the cuspids are as yet incomplete. The crowns of the first molars are near their completion, but the second molar is somewhat less advanced than the cuspids.

The process of the growth and absorption of the alveoli is interesting. It is first built up to enclose the teeth in process of formation. They erupting, it is absorbed to admit of the passage of their crowns. It is now rebuilt, to firmly secure the teeth in position. In the eruption of the permanent set it is again absorbed and rebuilt to form their sockets.

The process of dentition is a normal one, and should take place without any unpleasant or dangerous symptoms; but there are few children who pass through this period without suffering in a greater or less degree.

The teeth vary a great deal in their time of eruption, as regards different individuals. A premature eruption of them is much more liable to result in some disturbance, than if their eruption is retarded.

The teeth erupt in groups, The first group appear about seven months after birth, and consist of the two inferior central incisors.

Next come the four superior incisors at nine or ten months, and constitute the second group.

Now comes quite a long interval.

The next teeth to erupt are the two inferior lateral incisors and the four first molars, at from twelve to fifteen months. They are the third group.

The fourth group consists of the four cuspids, which appear from the eighteenth to the twenty-fourth month.

The fifth and last group includes the remaining teeth, the four second molars, and erupt from thirty to thirty-six months.

It has been a matter of some dispute as to whether the cuspids or the first molars are the cause of the most disturbance. The cuspids are the only ones that come in between two others. Mortality tables show that one out of every five infants dies before reaching the age of twelve months; and one out of every three children dies during the first five years of its life.

Now, out of this number, it has been asserted that over four per cent. of those dying during the first year that death was caused from diseases or affections resulting from dental irritation, and that seven per cent. of the deaths occuring between the ages of one and three years were from the same cause. It is thought, however, by later writers and practitioners that this is much exaggerated.

The causes of a deranged dentition are numerous.

The general health of the infant plays a very important part.

Physicians, as a rule, do not give the study and attention to the diseases of children that the subject demands, while a large proportion of their practice is among them.

The great predisposing cause of a disordered dentition is of course a lowered vitality of the system. Feeble children are more likely to suffer than robust ones. Living in crowded cities, where the atmosphere is always more or less vitiated, food in insufficient quantity or of inferior quality, must not be overlooked as predisposing causes, and it is very necessary that they should be corrected. Cleanliness is also of great importance. It is very necessary that the child be properly clothed. On the other hand, a child may be overfed, and experience evil results from that cause.

Too particular care should not be taken of children. A new born babe may be taken out in the air for several hours a day if the weather admits of it.

There seems to be no doubt that the process of dentition is charged with more mischief than is due to it. There are various affections which may be, and often are due to it; but may all be produced from some other cause.

In the infant the nervous system predominates, The salivary glands are comparatively inactive and do not secrete saliva proper. Perfect saliva is secreted at about three months. The child cannot digest starchy food until this period. The alimentary canal is comparatively shorter in the child. It is best to wean a child between the period of eruption of the second and third groups of teeth—ten or twelve months. It may begin to take solid food when teething commences, and when weaned let it be done somewhat gradually.

The secretions of the skin in infancy are extremely active; and from a lack of control of the sebaceous secretions, we have the occurrence of many skin diseases.

An erysipelatous mother should not nurse her child. A syphilitic mother may.

In the infant the stomach is small and straight, it is simply a dilation of the alimentary canal. It is not suited to retain food long, and the digestion is quick. The developement of the alimentary canal keeps pace with the teeth.

Rachitis, or more familiarily, rickets, is a condition of the system that much interferes with dentition. Its treatment is mostly hygienic, tonics probably are indicated.

Tubercule does not interfere with dentition. The alveolar ridges of the jaws may be small and unusually porous. There may be a lack of the proper amount of process, while it may still be normally compact. In these cases the anterior surfaces of the teeth can be felt through the gums. In the latter case dentition is easy. The irritation of an emptying tooth may disappear for a time and then return. This, perhaps, is caused by the resistance of the process first and then the resistance of the soft parts. The cases are rare where there is irritation from advancing teeth, and no local indications of it exist.

The dental difficulty itself may be but a symptom. The irritation from dentition may cause:

1. A stomatitis.
2. Irritative fevers.
3. Spasms.
4. Eruptions of the skin—especially of the scalp and face.

In the first of these (stomatitis) the inflammation may be a localized or diffused one, depending upon the degree of irritation, and the susceptibility of the child to such impression.

The first symptoms are an uneasy, itching sensation of the gums, an increased flow of saliva and tumefaction of the gums.

Now comes the question as to whether the lancet shall be used. If the child seems otherwise healthy, the swelling over the advancing tooth presents a glistening tense appearance, it is advisable to use the lancet in cases of the incisor teeth cutting in the direction of the arch, in the molars, making a crucial incision. A proper position for the patient and operator to be in, is to have the child sit upon the nurses lap with its face towards hers; the operator sitting facing the nurse, draws the head and body of the child backwards, and has then good control of it.

The gum lancet though often serving an excellent purpose, is an instrument not nearly so much in demand as in the past. Not only is its use not indicated, but it often aggravates the difficulty it is intended to relieve. Palliative treatment is preferable. Tincture of Belladonna, or a saturated solution of Potassium Bromide applied to the gums, will often suffice.

A little sack of ice held in the mouth will frequently give much relief. When the lance is used a cicatrix may form over the tooth which is more resistant than before the cutting. Hemorrhage is seldom troublesome after the proper use of the lance. If the bleeding is too profuse, mild astringents may be used, and internal medicament also.

The sucking propensity of infants is to be guarded against by the insertion of some article in the mouth to prevent its being able to form a vacuum. The dental irritation may be but the exciting cause of the disturbance, and only a small part of the treatment will therefore be directed to the teeth. Inflammation of the mouth may extend by continuity to the various parts lined by mucous membrane, or the irritation may excite a morbid action in almost any organ in the body.

The febrile state is perhaps the most frequent results of a disordered dentition. There is usually more or less fever. It is remarkable for the sudden rise and declination often. It is attended with much restlessness. The sleep is broken, thirst is great, and the appetite impaired. Our diagnosis will sometimes be difficult, we must look for causes aside from the teeth. Our treatment will be governed by the indications presented, though the same general treatment will be applicable to a majority of the cases. Refrigerating drinks are often very soothing and beneficial. Emetics and cathartics may be used with good effect. Potassium Bromide is often invaluable. If our treatment be not successful, we must look to discover if there are any surrounding or outside influences.

Diarrhœa so frequently occurring in the infant, is perhaps not as often the result of dental irritation as is generally supposed. The mucous membrane of the mouth, being continous with the orsophagus, stomach and intestines, it will be seen that an inflammation at one point may cause the whole tract to become irritable. Food in excess or of improper quality, worms, Enteritis. Tabes Mesenterica are among the causes of diarrhœa. Diarrhœa occurs more frequently in hot weather. The milk of a nurse is sometimes the cause of a diarrhœa. The nursing bottle is often in an unwholesome condition. After discovering if possible and removing the cause, medicines will often hasten the restoration to the normal condition. A long list of medicines have been resorted to for the relief of diarrhœa. Opium is perhaps one of the best. The administration of sweet oil and paregoric is a good form for the child; or small doses of Dover's powder. The citrate and tartrate of Potassium are also serviceable. Warm applications to the abdomen are often of good service. If the diarrhœa is not inflammatory in character the Bromide is indicated.

Spasms should here receive some notice. It is considered a direct or indirect irritation of the spinal cord or its branches. Here perhaps a little more liberty in lancing the gums will be allowed. We may cut down upon teeth whose period of erruption is at hand. It is good practice to insert into the incision made, a pledget of cotton saturated with a solution of sulphate of morphia. If the child is anaemic, tonics are indicated in connection with sedatives. If the child is plethoric, Potassium Bromide and the salines are indicated.

All stimulating food should be avoided. Hot foot baths will often be of service The abstraction of blood by leeches, or opening a vein may be necessary.

Spasm usually requires speedy relief. A babe in convulsion may be immersed in a warm bath of 75 degrees. Emetics which are not depressing should be used to rid the stomach of any undigested food. Chloral Hydrate is of great value, and if necessary, chloroform may be given to the babe.

I am unable to say to what extent the irritation of teething affects the skin. It is accountable for a share of such affections. Its consideration would make a long paper of itself. Dental irritation does not produce any skin diseases peculiar to that cause.

IRREGULARITIES.

Irregularity in the position of the temporary teeth is almost wholly confined to the incisors, particularly of the lower jaw. It is not generally advisable to interfere with them, unless they cause a bad articulation. Irregularity in the number of the temporary teeth is occasionally met with. Occasionally the jaws are entirely edentulous. I know one instance where this is the case with a woman and two or three of her children, who have now arrived at adult age. I have not yet had an opportunity of examining their mouths. I am at a loss to know how such cases can be accounted for. The jaws which contain more than the usual number, however, possess more practical interest. Supernumerary teeth do not usually resemble in form any of the natural teeth—their crowns are often conical. Cases have occurred, however, where they contributed to form a perfect arch, it being difficult to determine which was the extra tooth. If supernumerary teeth interfere with a proper articulation—if in a position which renders the jaws or lips unsightly, are annoying to the possessor, or are useless, they should be removed.

Fusion of the temporary teeth, which occurs in some instances, seems to be confined to the incisors and cuspids. It is caused by the union of the soft parts before calcification. They may be united by their crowns, roots, or nearly or all of the length of the tooth. It possesses but little practical interest, except that it has to be dealt with as one tooth. When they are attached only by the roots, it may not be discovered until one of them requires removal.

Inflammations of the tooth pulp should be treated in the same manner as in the permanent teeth.

When it becomes necessary to destroy the pulp of a temporary tooth, it being exposed, it is a dangerous and objectionable practice to use arsenic as the agent. The pulp may be touched a few times with Monsel's solution of iron or the tincture of iodine.

Saving the pulps alive, if possible, I believe preferable to devitalizing them, as dead teeth are more likely to become diseased in the child than the adult.

Abscesses connected with the temporary teeth may be looked upon with some alarm. If they do not yield speedily to treatment, or depend for their continuance on some constitutional cause, extraction is advisable. The greater susceptibility of the child, and the protection of the germs of the permanent teeth, render prompt relief necessary.

It will of course be admitted that cleanliness of the child's mouth is very important. The child should early be taught the use of the brush. Its teeth should be brushed for it before it is able to perform that little act of cleanliness for itself. After awhile it will not be objectionable to the child, on account of the more agreeable feeling produced in the mouth. Floss silk should be substituted for the toothpick, as it does its work far better. Such care would serve to prevent the deposition of green stain, so common to the teeth of children, and prevent a large share of decay.

I am unable to say what teeth of the temporary set are most commonly the seat of caries—probably the first molars, then the central incisors.

I think it is evident that there is much more harm done to the permanent set by the premature loss of the deciduous teeth than by the latter remaining too long. When the temporary molars are lost early, the tendency is for the first permanent molar to come forward in the mouth somewhat, thus giving less room for the anterior teeth. If the temporary teeth remain good until the proper time for their departure, it gives the jaws a better opportunity to expand and develop properly.

We occasionally find one or more of the deciduous teeth remaining until an advanced age. Whether it is their presence that prevents the eruption of the permanent teeth that should be their successors I know not; they should not, at least. Their successors, however, may sometimes never be formed. Carious temporary teeth should not be left in such condition for other reasons than their own preservation. They are injurious to the general health, and promote decay of the permanent teeth with which they are in contact.

Superficial decay, especially on the approximal surface of the teeth, may be removed by the use of the saw, the file, dia mond disk, and polishing with emory paper or cloth. Where the teeth are crowded it is good practice to separate them, and thus prevent the decay by affording a better opportunity for cleanliness. Such cavities that cannot be obliterated in this way should be filled. Of the various filling material now in use, it is difficult to say what would serve the best purpose in the greatest number of cases. It depends on the circumstances of the case—as to what tooth is to be filled, the location of the cavity in the tooth, the extent of the cavity, the length of time moisture can be kept from the cavity, etc. The disposition of the child will have much to do with making the operation a success or a failure, and it will often be found very trying to do anything for them at all.

I suppose all metallic fillings will preserve the teeth better where they are in a position in the tooth where the conditions are most uniform as regards moisture. Gold is used to a small extent, and there are some instances where it would surpass all other materials. In small cavities, its conducting property would not render it a source of irritation, and in a position in a tooth where it is observable, it presents a better appearance than any of the other metals. The difficulty of its insertion in many cavities is evident. Its good qualities I need not dwell upon.

Lead and tin are often of great value. Either of them may suffer from the action of the fluids of the mouth. The principal recommendation for lead is its adaptability and poor conducting power. Tin is to be considered with more favor. It possesses the good quality of being harder than lead and better able to resist chemical action. Tin, in the form of foil or felt, is quite easily introduced, and the operation much more speedy than with gold. Its conducting power is much less than gold, but on account of its being non-cohesive it cannot be retained in all cavities.

Amalgam should not be thought of in connection with the deciduous teeth. Hill's Stopping and Gutta Percha are admirable preparations, and will sometimes remain almost perfect for years in a tooth, it depending very much upon the location of the filling in the tooth.

The cements in the market are frequently of excellent service; withstanding the wear and the secretions of the mouth for a considerable period. Some of them are less irritating than others, and the operator should select the one suited to the case in hand.

The non-conducting property of guta percha and the cements render them very valuable in many cases. Here, as in the permanent teeth, the cements afford a good preparation to use in the bottoms of cavities which extend to near the pulp, or are especially sensitive while introducing the filling. The various agents for obtunding the sensitiveness of dentine used in the permanent teeth will be applicable here.

DISCUSSION OF THE TREATMENT OF DECIDUOUS TEETH.

Dr. Barrett.—The one principle that particularly underlies the salvation of deciduous teeth, and at the same time the one most embarrassing circumstance to be met, is the treatment of the pulp of these teeth. The process which nature has provided for the removal of these teeth is by the absorption of the roots, and the following of the permanant teeth through underneath them. The question therefore arises, are the roots of the deciduous teeth absorbed in cases where the pulps are dead? It has been asserted that they are, and also that they are not. I think Dr. Brophy has studied the pathology of this class of cases considerably, and I would like to hear his views upon that subject.

Dr. Brophy.—In my opinion teeth which have lost their vitality are incapable of being absorbed. They may become disintegrated the same as any of the osseous tissues. The cementum may lose its form by a process which we call caries or necrosis, and the dissolved calcium salts may find exit, or possibly be taken up. We know that bones are frequently lost through necrosis followed by liquefaction and gradual absorption until there is no bony structure left. It has been said that it is impossible for nature to remove a dead part by absorption. That I think is not true, because we know our bodies are being constantly repaired and renewed and replaced, the old tissues being absorbed. I think then that the roots of deciduous teeth, when devoid of vitality, are liquefied, as in cases of necrosis, gradually broken down and taken away by the absorbents. We know that in such cases as were mentioned this morning, the teeth are often deflected from the proper direction on one side or the other, and are liable to tip out. We find cases where the apex of the temporary tooth is turned out through the gum. That would show that the pressure of the permanent tooth is not sufficient to produce the absorption necessary to removal.

There are other matters pertaining to the treatment of deciduous teeth that I might speak of. Sometimes decay commences as early, in the incisors, as the first or second year. I think the better way to treat these cases is simply to separate the teeth by means of a file, cutting them so they may be free, in the manner recommended by Dr. Arthur. This insures a thorough cleansing. With the teeth of my own children, where caries has commenced, I have resorted to that method myself. One little girl, now seven years old, had carries commence between the central incisors when she was about a year and a half old. I made free separations at that time, and the teeth are no more diseased than they then were. There is some caries, but the teeth still remain. The great point is to get them so that they will cleanse themselves freely. Now, as to filling cavities in the teeth, the pulps of which are alive, I have good success in using guta percha. I have also used amalgam, but I have objections to that. Tin or phosphate of zinc are excellent materials, where the cavity can be thoroughly cleansed and dried. In cases where deciduous molars are somewhat decayed, I would pursue the same treatment, making free cuts, so that the apex of the V shaped cut will be at the bottom, and the broad base at the top, in lower teeth and vice versa in the upper. I speak only of the temporary teeth in those cases. It is a very important point that a systematic brushing of the teeth should be begun very young.

Dr. Hunter.—In cases where you think there is perhaps some absorption, or something of that nature of a deciduous tooth, after the death of the nerve, is that analagous to absorption as naturally performed. Then, again, with reference to the absorption of bones in the other parts of the body. Do you know of any cases which you have seen or read of where the periosteum of the bone has been destroyed, and the necrosis takes place in which the dead matter is carried off by absorption, as you call it? True absorption, as we understand it, is a symmetrical process, and I do not consider the apparent absorption after the death of the nerve, as anything except necrosis.

DR. BROPHY—As I understand it is a case of necrosis, followed by the excretion of the liquefied substance in the same manner that other dead substances are carried away.

DR. HUNTER.—I refer to cases where the part becomes necrosed and the periosteum dead, not where there is simply a shrinking away for want of nourishment or something of that kind.

DR. BROPHY.—Usually when necrosis of the bone takes place, fistuluous openings are formed through which the liquefied substance, the fine granules of calsium, which compose the bone, are thrown out, but that is not always the case. Sometimes a part will be gone, will have wholly disapeared, without the fistulous openings having formed or any external appearance taking place, but where the dead matter has been carried away through the action of the absorbents.

DR. HARROUN.—Each individual practioner is supposed to be endowed with a certain amount of intelligence, (and he is expected to use this intelligence) for the benefit of the patient. Our practice in any particular case must, it seems to me, be governed very largely by the conditions which exist in that particular case. It is a very difficult matter to classify all the cases which come under our notice. We should be guided by the symptoms and conditions of the individual, and thus be able to determine intelligently whether the treatment should be internal and general, or local to the teeth. I agree as to the treatment of separating decayed temporary teeth as much as practicable from the permanent ones. This will allow thorough cleansing. In a good many cases, however, owing to local difficulties, I would not do that. I have pursued this practice in my own family, but I have had cases where I could not control the patients, or get them to follow my directions as to subsequent treatment. Parents of patients themselves often think that if the teeth of their children are filled, that is all the attention which is necessary to give to them. This makes it difficult to carry out any line of treatment as we would like to. Parents should be taught to keep the teeth of their children cleaned, and especially at bed time, if they would preserve them from decay and abcess of the nerve. As to the filling that should be used, it depends very much upon the structure of the tooth. Guta percha can be used where nothing harder would do. I have been using tin foil a great deal, and find it very successful. It has a peculiar chemical condition different from most other minerals, and I like it very well.

Dr. Clawson.—In regard to deciduous teeth I wish to speak from my own experience. I have a little girl, now seven years old. I began caring for her teeth and brushing them just as soon as she would hold her mouth open and allow me to do it. She now has all of her first teeth, with no sign of irregularity or decay. These teeth are not extremely hard, they are only ordinary in that respect. I use a preparation partly of chalk. I did use the clear powdered chalk.

In regard to devitalized temporary teeth I cannot be convinced but what the membrane can be restored by proper treatment. Dr. Talbot spoke as though he thought there was no absorption of the roots, but I cannot see why it could not be done if we can remove the nerve or pulp from the cavity, and leave the membrane around the root in a healthy condition. I think the membrane is very apt to be stronger if properly treated after the death of the pulp, and I think it performs the work of the pulp.

Dr. Harlan—We are all aware that the absorption of the roots of deciduous teeth is a physiological process; that there is an absorbent papilla in connection with the root and over the tooth that is absorbed. If the papilla of the tooth has been destroyed it is not possible that true absorption follows. In other words it would seem that the absorption of a pulpless deciduous tooth is not possible. Another error that has formed a part of some of this discussion is that the incoming tooth produces absorption. I think there is no gentleman present who has not seen an incisor, particularly of the permanent set, come in inside or outside of a deciduous tooth. This would show that no absorption has taken place. That one fact pretty clearly demonstrates that it is not pressure which produces absorption, because in instances of that kind where the permanent tooth forces its way through on one side of the temporary tooth or the other, there is a great amount of pressure. The late Dr. Dean, of Chicago, has investigated that process perhaps as thoroughly as anyone, and his conclusions are something like what I have stated. There can be no absorption; that there is liquefaction I believe. Dr. Spaulding of St. Louis claims that he has filled the roots of deciduous teeth with gold, and afterwards found the little spiculæ of gold projecting into the soft surrounding surface without irritation when he extracted the teeth. He is the only one who has ever claimed that. No one else has ever contributed anything to the literature of the treatment of deciduous teeth analagous to it. I shall not dispute it, but I should like to see it. Now, if the pulp of a deciduous molar tooth be destroyed at six years of age and the root filled, the tooth being extracted a year or two later, there would undoubtedly be an excavation in some one of the roots, which would show that there had been absorption; but that absorption would have taken place previous to the destruction of the pulp. As in fractures of the maxillæ, and other accidents, where teeth have been knocked out at those stages, the results of absorption can be seen. It is thus demonstrated that the process of absorption begins very early, as early as the sixth year in the first temporary molars.

As to the filling of deciduous teeth with gutta percha, I wish to say this: I have experimented with every form of gutta percha that has been manufactured, I think, in the United States, England or France. The best that I have found for working purposes is Jackob's gutta percha, manufactured in England. It is superior on account of its finer grain, and its resistance to friction. Its qualities are such that it is possible to work more rapidly with it, filling a tooth in a very few minutes at the outside. It is very expensive, costing I think, about ten dollars an ounce, but that is no objection if you desire to save the teeth.

Dr. Taft.—In the paper which has been read there are several points which have been referred to. I will speak of one, the shedding of the temporary teeth. This has been spoken of as a physiological process, and it undoubtedly is when health in the parts has been maintained. It is accomplished by the dissolving of the dentine of the roots, beginning at the end and sometimes upon the side of the root. It is a dissolving and not a liquefaction. The use of that term has been rather inappropriate. The liquefaction of a substance is a transition from a solid to a fluid state. Take a piece of ice for instance. By the application of heat it is liquefied. Dissolving is simply bringing a substance in contact with another substance that will transform it from a solid to a fluid state. For example, a piece of sugar is brought into contact with its proper solvent and is dissolved. When we say that the root of a tooth has been liquefied it gives the idea that it has been simply transformed from a solid to a liquid state, without the intervention of any other immediate substance or material.

In a healthy state the roots of the teeth are dissolved away, nature furnishing an arrangement for the process. There is a new tooth being formed, and usually below the temporary tooth, sometimes on the side, but between the newly formed permanent tooth and the temporary tooth, there is a little body or organ denoted variously; Harris denoting it as the "carneous body," a dissolving organ which nature puts there just as any other organ of the body is formed for a purpose. It has a work to perform. The function of that little fleshy mass is to elaborate a material that will dissolve the root away where it comes in contact with it. As the new tooth grows and the temporary one is dissolved away, this little fleshy mass simply passes up and is borne upon the crown of the growing permanent tooth, and kept in contact with the temporary tooth which is being dissolved off. This little fleshy body is not a peculiar form of the pulp of the temporary tooth, as has been asserted by some high authorities. That this is not true is shown by the fact that the process goes on while the pulp of the temporary tooth remains, or part of it at least. The material that is dissolved from the end of the root is taken up and disposed of through the system as any other debris or material would be. This process goes on and by and by the pulp of the temporary tooth is destroyed. This will take place perhaps at various periods during the time of this wasting away of the end of the root. Our observation will, I think, bear out the truth of the presentation which I make here. By and by it is found there is no pulp in the crown at all, that it is gone, and yet after that the root continues to be dissolved away, if this little fleshy body is brought against the roots. Sometimes this wasting away of the roots occurs upon the side of the tooth. Where this is found, the little body between the root of the temporary tooth and the crown of the permanent tooth is against the side of the tooth; and so the process goes on in the same way. Remove the temporary tooth a little time before it is ready to be taken away, and there you will find this little pinkish red pulpy mass lying between the crown of the advancing permanent tooth and the nearly dissolved root of the temporary tooth.

But the question has been sometimes asked, "If the action of this little body dissolves off the roots of the temporary tooth, why does it not dissolve the enamel of the crown of the permanent tooth beneath it?" The reason is that it only throws out the dissolving material from the side next to the root of the temporary tooth. This is a normal and physiological process, but very frequently there is more or less disease, and this must be taken into account.

The question has been raised, "Do the roots of pulpless temporary teeth ever become dissolved away?" Yes; they do become dissolved away, even though the pulp may have been destroyed whenever this little body below has not become deteriorated by the debris of the decomposing pulp. If this little tissue, which is in the main independent of the pulp of the temporary tooth, retains its integrity, in a healthy condition, it will go on dissolving away the ends of the temporary teeth, no matter whether the pulp is there or not. But the result would be, in a great majority of cases, that the debris resulting from the death of the pulp would be sufficient to produce disease in, or wholly destroy this little body, and so prevent its further working for dissolution of the roots. I think it is uniformally true that in all cases where inflammation takes place, the function of this body is either very seriously impaired, or entirely destroyed.

But are the roots of temporary teeth sometimes dissolved away, even under such circumstances as this? Yes; and sometimes the roots of permanent teeth are dissolved away. They are sometimes honey-combed; they are sometimes dissolved more or less at the end. Occasionally I have seen one-half of the root of a permanent tooth dissolved away, though not by the same process as a temporary tooth is dissolved. By a diseased condition in which the elaboration of a solvent takes place the root is dissolved away. The same thing takes place with the temporary teeth, but it is a natural physiological action, and not the process that takes place upon the roots of permanent teeth where a sinus forms around them.

As to the treatment of temporary teeth I wish to say a few words. We cannot understand the management of them, or of any other organs of the body unless we know the natural physiological processes, as well as the pathological, which attach to them. So it is the very foundation of our knowledge in regard to the management of the temporary teeth, to know how they come in, what they do, and how the different processes that attach to them takes place, as well as the instrumentalities by which they take place, so far as we can understand them. We have taken things for granted too much. We cannot understand many of these things, but we do live and learn and we can all improve. The permanent teeth are influenced somewhat by the forces and processes which act at about the period when the roots of the temporary teeth are taken away. A temporary tooth may have a serious effect sometimes upon the permanent tooth which succeeds it. Sometimes the crown of a permanent tooth will appear with the enamel roughened all over its surface, and sometimes almost dissolved. Sometimes you can scrape off the enamel it is so nearly dissolved. These conditions are always due to the failure in the developing process. This carneous body is diseased and its utility perverted, or destroyed altogether. The crown of the permanent tooth therefore comes in contact with the root of the temporary tooth, and so this roughening occurs.

In regard to the removal of the temporary teeth, I think it is a subject well worthy of our thought. The proper period for the removal of the temporary teeth is a serious question. A temporary tooth, if its roots are not dissolved away, should be taken away at the time of the appearance of the crown of the permanent tooth.

Dr. Barrett—I am of the opinion that this little papilla which has been spoken of must necessarily be a gland. It cannot be anything else according to the Doctor's own description of it. It must be a gland because it secretes something, and if it be a gland it must be connected with the glandular system. Now, it seems to me, that leads you into an error, an absurdity. According to the Doctor's way of arguing it cannot be anything but a gland. I am speaking now according to the nomenclature of it, or according to the histology of it. I do not subscribe to the Doctor's theory at all. There are three schools of histology, the English, German and French. I suppose if we were to ask the question, as to what this process is, if we were to put it to an English histologist, he would say it is a kind of necrosis. A German histologist, like Virchow, might say it was a solution of some kind. A Frenchman would say it was a return to embryonal condition, and I think our friend Atkinson would say that. Robin and Pouchet would assert, I think, that it is a return to embryonal condition. Which of these theories we choose does not matter particularly, but I cannot understand that by any possible theory has it ever been demonstrated, or can it be, that there is any separate, special, individual organ whose office is the removal of the tooth by solution. Any substance which has such power as to effect the solution of the tooth must be as powerful as most of the strong acids are. Now, if this be so then the absorption of the permanant teeth would probably be effected in the same manner, and would require another special creation of a special organ for a special purpose to last for a definite and specified time, and then be removed. I do not understand that such is the case. My idea is that it is a particular physiological process, not of one organ which has but this one definite office to perform. It returns again to something which might be called embryonal conditions and may even be restored into new matter again. New corpuscles can be formed through the formation of nuclei. This word embryonal conditions, although it does not express exactly my own idea, is the expression which Robin uses. I wish to get a general expression of opinion upon the subject of the absorption or resorption of the deciduous teeth. I wish to get at what the general idea of it is, whether it is by solution, through the action of a fluid sufficiently strong and powerful to dissolve away the organic matter of the tooth, or what the process is. I wish to know, too, what the idea is as to how this matter is carried away. It requires a vascular supply in order that it shall be carried away, and that must be from the glandular system. It is carried into the blood, and not simply deposited.

DR. TAFT—That is where it goes.

DR. BARRETT—But here we have this definite corpuscle, this carneous body, of which you speak, which must be a gland. It cannot be confined to that—to the office of dissolution, it must be a secretive body. If this be true then what becomes of the solution that is carried into the circulation?

DR. TAFT—Is it not possible that this body performs a double function, elaboration of the solvent, and then the disposing of the matter dissolved.

DR. BARRETT—Do you know of any instance anywhere in the human body where any one organ has these two functions or anything approaching them? I know of nothing analogous to it in the human system. I cannot subscribe to Professor Taft's theory. I believe this process to be a physiological one and not a breaking down of the tooth.

DR. TAFT—Is it carried away in particles without being dissolved, or does solution take place?

DR. BARRETT—That is what Virchow would say. I believe it is a part of a physiological process of nature, returning the material back to the matter from which it was constructed in the first place, back to a condition of nature, the pabulim of the cells. I do not mean exactly that, but a condition very nearly analogous to it, so that there may be formed new material; what the French school calls a re-secretion by means of epiblasts. I do not subscribe to that theory altogether, but still it is something of that kind. Now what becomes of all the effected matter thrown off by the human system, by the tissues, the whole being taken away. Surely it is not disposed of by means of any special process, but it is a part of the general process dependent upon the circulation. There is a return to a condition where it can be taken up by the absorbents.

DR. TAFT—Certainly.

Dr. Barrett—It is not by any special organ.

The idea so very frequently expressed in all the medical works that the eruption of the teeth, during the period of dentition, causes such irritation and derangement of the whole digestive system, is I think, an erroneous one. In health the eruption of the teeth is a perfectly physiological process. It should no more effect the general condition of the system than the growing of one's hair or finger nails. It is entirely physiological. Why is it then that people are particularly liable to stomach diseases just at that time. Because it is between hay and grass with the child, to use a common expression. It is just at the time when the digestive organs are undergoing a change from that simple diet and pabulum for which they were adapted in the first place, to a grosser, heavier diet. During this change children are peculiarly liable to stomatitis and difficulties of that kind. This is not caused by the eruption of the teeth. It comes from mal-nutrition, indigestion or something of that kind. The irritation caused by the erruption of the teeth has nothing more to do with it than the growing of the hair upon one's head. I believe that there is a hundred times more injury done by the cutting of the gums than by leaving them alone. If the child is in anything like a healthy state there is no trouble about his teething. When there is sufficient pressure upon the gums there will be absorption of the gums, and the tooth will come through easily. In cutting the gums nineteen times out of twenty, and I don't know but oftener, it is done at the wrong time and a cicatricial tissue is formed which only increases the difficulty in the eruption of the teeth. If I ever did cut the gums at all, I should slip the point of a pen-knife under the gums and cut upwards and outwards; I have seen children that were extremely ill, nearly in convulsions. I remember one particular case where I felt very confident that the cutting of the gums would relieve the difficulty, because of the extreme tension existing in the gums. I had read so much about the pressure producing convulsions. So I cut the gums, but it did not do any good. It was simply a case of stomatitis, indigestion or gastritis. The cutting of the gums was not of the slightest benefit to the child.

Dr. Hunter—It has been remarked that the eruption of the teeth was a perfectly physiological process. I would like to ask if the transition from a lighter to a heavier diet, which the doctor has spoken of, is not also a perfectly physiological process, as much so as the eruption of the teeth.

Dr. Barrett—Not by a great deal.

Dr. Hunter—I can see it in no other light, doctor.

Dr. Whiting—when I began dentistry we had not the aids which our younger brethren have to-day in the way of Dental Colleges. We had to work out conclusions for ourselves. After I had been practicing dentistry about a year I thought I knew a great deal more about it than my preceptor did. The first case that I had, where a child's teeth were troubling it, I learned a great deal. Before that I had thought I knew more than all God's creation. The child was crying when brought to my office. I wisely passed my finger into its mouth and finding a little lump in the gum I lanced it, and almost immediately the child went to sleep. I got a great deal of credit for that operation. About a week after that a tooth came through nicely about an inch from where I had cut the gum. This led me to believe that the cutting of that gum did not amount to shucks. I believe that when a child is suffering in this condition, it is more of a disarranged condition of the stomach than it is from local irritation. A warm bath, a gentle rubbing with the hand will produce quietness quicker than blood letting of the gums, and be more beneficial. The local irritation ceases when the general circulation is increased.

Dr. Brophy—I have been very much interested and amused at the course the discussion has taken. I disagree entirely with what Dr. Barrett has said in regard to lancing of the gums. Furthermore I am surprised that he should state, as a physiologist, that the breaking through a cicatricial tissue is far more difficult than breaking through ordinary tissues. A cicatrice in all cases is the most easy and yielding of any. A cut which has healed is a great deal more yielding than the original tissue. Even if the gums do heal up and a cicatrice forms, cut them again and relieve the parts of the blood which has accumulated and which brings about this disturbance. I am convinced that the pressure upwards, by the teeth against the tissues produces a disturbance of the nervous system, and that is what brings about the trouble. That this simple operation on the gums has been productive of a great deal of good and saved the lives of hundreds of children, I have not a particle of doubt. I do it in my own family, and have often done it in other cases. Very frequently the child has fallen asleep, just as the one did that Dr. Whiting spoke of. It is not what is done so much as having done something to take away the congested blood which has produced the disturbance.

I desire here to correct a phrase that is used frequently in dental associations. Lime and the lime salts have been spoken of as forming a part in the teeth. This use of this word is wholly improper.

Dr. Taft—We use the expression carbonate of lime and phosphate of lime.

Dr. Brophy—There is no such thing as the carbonate of lime or the phosphate of lime in the teeth. I think I will convince you that that is true. Lime is the oxide of calcium, and I say there is no oxide of calcium in the tooth. The tooth is made up of the carbonate of the oxide of calcium, and not the oxide of calcium or the carbonate of calcium. To speak of the oxide, the carbonate, the flouride, etc. is improper. I think the paper read spoke of the use of lead in filling teeth. I was not aware that lead is now used for that purpose.

Dr. Barrett—I think the doctor's criticism upon the use of the expression carbonate of lime is a little far fetched. It is a perfectly common term, and as such I think the use is justifiable.

I cannot subscribe to the idea of curing congestion by lancing the gums and thus removing all the difficulties connected with dentition. If you are going to lance the gums for the sake of the bleeding I will agree with you; but as to performing this operation as a cure for stomatitis, gastritis, etc., I do not agree with that. The trouble has its origin back of the inflammation and irritation in these diseases and disarrangements of the stomach which produce convulsions and death itself in some cases.

Dr. Whiting—I wish to relate one experience more which is pertinent to this discussion. A few days after this success of mine that I spoke of, I was called to see a child that was cutting its teeth in the same way. The child was cross and would not let me look into its mouth. The mother gave the child a good spankimg and it went to sleep just as quickly as the one whose gums I had lanced.

Dr. Douglass—For twenty-five years I have not cut a child's gums in consequence of suffering from teething, as it is called, in but two cases. These two cases were where physicians sent the children to me and I did not feel at liberty to prescribe any other treatment. I cut the gums in accordance with the request of the physicians. It is a practice however that I am opposed to. I believe it is erroneous and the sooner the profession entirely discontinue it the better it will be for us, and the better will be our credit. I have had the treatment of a good many cases and my experience has led me to come to this conclusion. Where the child's digestive organs are in a proper condition, and the child if furnished with proper food in the proper amount, I do not think it ever suffers from teething to any great extent. If the food is not proper, or if it is given in excessive quantities, a disturbance will be produced.

As an example of what can be done by specific medication, I wish to relate a single instance. I was called to see a child about eight months old. It had been lying in an unconscious state for about five hours. I could not attract its attention in any way. The child could not swallow. The mouth was open and the tongue dry. The eyes were partly open and turned upward, the white of the eye congested, the head hot and the feet cold. The mother told me it had been suffering for several hours; that it had first cried continually and then went into this unconscious state. I put a few pellets medicated with a dilution of aconite, perhaps the second dilution upon the child's tongue. The result was astonishing to me. Since then I have learned not to be astonished by a good many repetitions of the same state of affairs. In a few moments I could see a change in the child. It began to move its eyes in different directions, instead of having them remain rolling up. In about eight minutes it looked up intelligently at the mother, looked at me, recognized me beyond any question, and began to move its hands. In ten minutes it reached out its hands for its little rattlebox. I then told the mother that if the child needed any further care to let me know. The next time I saw the mother she told me that within a few hours the child was apparently perfectly well. I am a believer in specific medication.

DR. BARRETT—Was the child suffering from a disease incident to teething?

DR DOUGLASS—Its gums were all swollen.

DR. BARRETT—Would it not have been well to have followed Hanemann's directions to allow the child to smell the cork of the bottle?

DR. DOUGLASS—Perhaps others can answer that question better than I can. I have known persons to be cured of neuralgia by inhaling aconite. I have no doubt in many cases that would be sufficient.

I wish to speak in regard to the roots of deciduous teeth, after the crowns are decayed so that the pulp has died. The process seems to be very much more rapid than with the roots of the permanent teeth. I have met with one instance where I was called upon to extract the root of a deciduous central incisor for a child only fourteen months old. There was only a very narrow portion of the gum remaining on the anterior surface of the root. The child manifested no indications of suffering. In regard to the proper time when it is necessary to remove such roots I make this a rule; if an abcess has formed and puss is discharging in such a quantity that it cannot be removed by internal or local treatment, I remove the root. If an abcess has formed and the inflammation has subsided so that the discharge is very light, I think it is best to leave the roots until pretty nearly the time for the new tooth to take its place. I do not agree exactly with the doctor who spoke about making a V-shaped cut between the second deciduous molar and the first permanent molar. I make the V-shaped space, but don't make the opening of the V toward the teeth on the opposite jaw. I would make it toward the teeth on the opposite side of the same jaw, partly, and partly carried back toward the teeth on the lower jaw. In this way the cavity will clear itself during the process of mastication and arrest decay. I have seen teeth which have been of service for a good many years after such an operation.

Dr. Brophy—It has always been my habit whenever I found an abcess with pus ready to be removed, to open it. It has been my habit also whenever I found blood congested in the vessels of the gums to relieve the congestion.

In reference to my criticism of the use of the expression lime salts, I have only this to say; that to speak of the chloride of calcium, the flouride of calcium, etc., does not make the expression right. Because these terms have been used for a long time that is no excuse why they should be used longer.

Dr. Taft—Indulge me in a word or two more in reference to what Dr. Barrett said about the removal of the roots of temporary teeth. It seems to me that it is performed in a certain way by a certain temporary arrangement of nature for that purpose, and it matters not what it is called. This temporary material does not exist before a certain period, and it does not exist after its work is performed. As to the process, I regard it as simply a solution, a dissolving by which the material is taken away. It goes somewhere, and is not a state of solution the easiest way for nature to carry it off? It is not a breaking off of pieces of the hard material, a process of exfoliation. The root is dissolved, a solution is effected. It is not a return to embryonal condition; that is simply embryonal nonsense.

Something has been said in regard to the decay of the teeth; that it was a return to the material of the structure in an embryonal condition. It seems to me that is simply an expression to cover up, "I don't know." It looks that way to me. I do not state positively that the theory which I have advanced is not a mistaken one, but certainly this is a fact that the organ I speak of is there. The work is accomplished in its presence and it is not accomplished while the organ is absent. That organ is borne against the root of the temporary teeth by the advance of the permanent teeth. In the absence of the permanent teeth the organ also is absent. This is the method, the instrumentality that accomplishes the work as it strikes me.

In regard to the treatment during the period of dentition, cases of difficult dentition have been referred to. It is from disturbed functions that the trouble arises. If the growing tooth comes as it should, and is properly supported in its growth, if the way is prepared for it as it advances there will be no difficulty in the way of dentition later. The difficulty is that there is a defect in nutrition, a disturbance of some sort. Usually the great difficulty is produced by pressure upon the nerves in the parts pressed upon. Now, I do not presume that the actual pressure of the tooth is the normal means of preparing its way. I think the normal process should be independent of the pressure of the teeth. I do not think the tooth struggles through the surrounding tissue. I think the tissue is absorbed away in anticipation of the coming of the tooth. The gum affords but little resistance when everything is in a healthy state, for by a physiological function the way is prepared. If there is any disturbance of this process then the tooth comes in contact with the tissue, and pressure is sometimes the result as we know. The irritation consequent upon the failure of this work of preparation may result in one of two ways. The pressure of the teeth may produce irritation and inflammation. The pressure in the blood vessels may operate to produce a nervous disturbance through the parts. That is one way in which pain is produced. Another way, and a more serious one as it seems to me, is when the pressure becomes greater, and the blood is forced out of the vessels. Then the pressure upon the parts is just the same or greater. In such cases as that there will be more frequent reflex nervous influence exhibited one way or the other, on the brain, the stomach, the digestive apparatus, the alimentary apparatus or some other. As to the treatment of these cases, I agree with Dr. Barrett in much that he has said concerning the cause of the trouble, and if there is time to remedy it, very well. On the other hand, here is a child in convulsions, or about to die with cerebral disturbance produced in that way. It is just an extremity. What is to be done? There is no time to give constitutional treatment, and something must be done or the child is gone. Then come in these treatments which have been referred to, lancing the gums, or almost anything that will relieve the pressure and cause the nervous influences to subside. Counter-irritation will sometimes relieve the disturbance at the point where there is the most congestion.

Another thing referred to was the objection to lancing the gums, on the ground that a cicatrice, if formed, would be more difficult to clear away than anything else. I do not believe it. I have never seen a cicatrice form upon a gum where it had been cut at anything like a reasonable time or where there was any occasion for it at all. I do not believe that a cicatricial tissue may be formed at any ordinary period when the gum should be separated by lancing. I have heard of it, and have been looking for an instance of that kind for the last forty years, but never have found it, and I do not think it would be any obstacle if it should occur. I think that the treatment by counter-irritation, by a mustard plaster upon the back of the neck, or something of that kind, will many times act just as promptly as the other; but it seems to me that this operation upon the gums is simply a rational one that can be easily understood, and that no one need make any mistake about.

Dr. Douglass—Where the gums are cut I do not think there is usually the formation of a cicatrice. I wish to make one more remark in reference to a case of extreme absorption of a deciduous tooth. I have seen an instance where not only the root, but more than half the crown was absorbed, where only a very thin portion of the tooth, only part of the length of the crown remained.

EVENING SESSION.

Dr. Taft. I have one point further upon which I wish to speak in reference to the care of the teeth, of a prophylactic character, and that is in regard to the use of the temporary teeth. I presume that in a great many instances they become diseased, and are many times lost, simply from not being used as they should be. From the time the teeth are cut they should be used as nature designed them to be used, for the mastication of food. They should be used sufficiently to give them proper exercise for their development, so that they may perform what nature intended they should accomplish. If the food given a child is of a soft character, that requires no exercise of the teeth, and this is habitually kept up, they become enfeebled, and are more easily attacked by disease of all sorts, not only in respect to decay, but the periostem becomes affected more or less, and the gums are far more likely to be affected than if the teeth are used sufficiently to give them strength and proper development. I think the difficulty arises many times from this kind of food that requires no mastication at all, the child being permitted to take the food into the mouth and swallow it without mastication. Sometimes the food is cut up and made into a bolus, under the mistaken impression on the part of the kind and loving mother that it is the best way. The food should be of a character to require mastication, not only for the sake of comminution, but for the proper salivation, and to give the exercise necessary to add strength and tone to the periosteal attachment. Then another thing; the friction of the teeth and the washing of the saliva will keep them clean. It is utterly impossible to make the use of the brush with a little child a very great success, and some other way must be devised. Of course the brush must be used occasionally, but that is not sufficient. Indeed, one cannot with the brush alone accomplish all that would be accomplished by the proper use of the teeth in mastication. This is a matter in which nurses and mothers should be educated.

Another important consideration is the giving of strength and expansion to the jaws. If the teeth are used as they should be, the jaw is expanded and the temporary teeth are separated when the age of five or six years is reached. When this is accomplished, you will ordinarily find very little difficulty in the way of decay of the temporary teeth. The inferior and upper teeth are separated from each other. There is thus plenty of room for the permanent teeth when they come. A very good illustration of the effect of this is found in the jaws of many tobacco chewers, which are usually much stronger than those of men who do not exercise their teeth in mastication. Chewing gum has much the same effect.

Dr. Whiting.—Dr. Taft has struck just what I meant to draw out in my remarks this morning. The exercise of the teeth is as important as the exercise of the arm. Why does the right arm of the blacksmith measure sixteen inches and the left arm only twelve? It is on account of the difference in the exercise which they get, and the same principle is involved in the development of the teeth. Where the teeth are not properly exercised, the difficulty does not end with them, but extends much further. By failing to use our teeth sufficiently we are lessening the use of our stomachs. I do not suppose there are half a dozen men in Detroit but what realize that they have stomachs. If the teeth were properly exercised, and the food properly prepared for digestion, no healthy person would need to know that he had a stomach. We want some one who will invent a system of dental gymnastics. We must have something of this kind if we would save our teeth.

DR. DOUGLASS.—The proper exercise of the teeth is beneficial in more than one way; not simply by the friction of the food against the teeth keeping them clean, but it causes an increased circulation of the blood through the jaws, thus carrying the proper nourishment for the teeth. The teeth are thus built up and developed. They become much harder and stronger. I am well satisfied that the habit of chewing hard substances, which do not come to pieces readily, is very beneficial to the teeth. The question has been asked about chewing gum. I am satisfied that my own teeth are better than they would have been if I had not chewed gum when I was a boy.

DR. HUNTER,—This association should be, among other things, an educator of the people with reference to their teeth. If a few simple facts could be instilled into the minds of those who have the care of children, it would relieve a great deal of ignorance that exists at the present time, and it would relieve us from spending a great deal of time in trying to have our patients understand how to take care of their teeth. It seems to me that some benevolently disposed member should present something to this association for general dissemination among the people. I make this as a suggestion merely.

DR. THOMAS.—I think the suggestion of Dr. Hunter is a good one, and it brings to my mind an action taken either by this or the National Association. Some years ago a committee was appointed to confer with the publishers of school books, and see if we could not get introduced into school readers some short, terse articles on the care of the teeth and the hygiene of the mouth.

DR. MOORE.—It was this association.

DR. THOMAS.—I think so. I have thought of that a great many times since, and wondered what came of it—whether any action was ever taken. It is less than a week ago that in consulting the school readers of my small children I was very much gratified to find some articles on hygiene, the like of which never appeared in the readers when I was a boy, twenty-five or thirty years ago. That is a step in the right direction. On seeing these articles it occurred to me that this matter had been discussed in some of our associations.

Dr. Hunter.—My recollection is that it was this association.

Dr. Thomas.—I think that is true, and I do really think that a good deal can be accomplished in this line. I do believe that if the proper committee were appointed, composed of men of large experience who would write short, terse articles on the care of the teeth, in such a way that they would entertain children, a great deal of good could be accomplished. This would be a great deal better than to fill our readers with so much trash and nonsense as they now contain. I do not believe, either, that it would be very much of a task to get publishers to introduce this. Books are being changed constantly, and it seems to me that the society which will take the initiatory step in this direction will be looked upon as entitled to a great deal of credit.

While Dr. Whiting was speaking, it occurred to me that we did not half appreciate the fact, many of us, that a proper exercise of the teeth is necessary, not only to the health of the teeth themselves, but of the stomach and all of the organs of the body. The other day, while making a call on a gentleman with whom I am well acquainted, I was invited into the kitchen to see a new machine that he had purchased for the cutting of beefsteak. The machine had been sold him by one of the hardware merchants in the city. You may, some of you have seen it. By means of a revolving set of knives, operated by levers, a piece of steak when put into the machine is, in a few moments, chopped into a fine mass, almost a jelly. Two or three years previous I had undertaken to make a set of teeth which would aid him in mastication, but had failed from the fact that he had lost his lower molars a great many years ago. He is now fifty years old, and the upper teeth had come down and dragged on the lower gum. I put in a plate, thinking that he might be able to grind on the plate, but the operation was not a success, and in a short time he cast the plate aside. He got this chopping machine to cut up his beefsteak. He said to me, "I have the start of you now, doctor; I have something that is better than all your artificial teeth for preparing my food." After witnessing its operation and tasting some of the beefsteak which was prepared in this way, and which certainly was delicious, requiring no mastication whatever, he asked me, "What do you think of it?" I said: Sir, I think in your case it may be a benefit; but I think it is the very worst thing you could have introduced into your family. I had had the care of his children for the last eight or ten years. I reminded him of that fact, and said to him, It has baffled all my skill—which is not very much—to attempt to save these children's teeth. His children's teeth were so frail and poor that one of his children, who was in my office only a short time ago, and is now fifteen years of age, has every tooth in her mouth filled. Some of them have five or six fillings in them, and they are going, going. This is only one of seven or eight children. He could not understand why it was, for his children were very much pleased with the machine and its results. He was very much surprised when I told him what I did, but I went on to explain that the food, when prepared in this way, needs no mastication, the saliva does not become incorporated with it, and it is swallowed whole, without being properly prepared for reception into the stomach. The children in this family are growing up like plants in a cellar, and it is very unfortunate that it is so. The man who deprives his children of their proper exercise, either of their teeth or the rest of their bodies, is doing them a positive harm. In this case it is not only the teeth, but the general systems of the children, that are weakened from a lack of exercise. One of them is scrofulously inclined, and when in my office, only a few days ago, she had her face all patched up. She has been under treatment for some years for glandular troubles, and it is largely owing, in my opinion, to the lack of exercise and proper development. I think Dr. Whiting's term, "dental gymnastics," is a good one. It is one that I have been needing for a long time. It looks in the right direction. I hope to see something done about this matter of the introduction of short articles on dental hygiene in our school books. It would be well to consider the question again.

MORNING SESSION.

DISCUSSION ON THE RELATION OF DENTISTRY TO MEDICINE.

(Dr McGregor's paper on this subject, printed in the proceedings of 1881, was read.)

DR. HAROUN.—A remark is made in the paper which we have just heard in reference to physicians not knowing as much as they ought to know always on the subject of the diseases which arise from imperfections of the teeth. This is sometimes lamentably the case. I know of at least one instance in which the want of proper knowledge on the part of the physician resulted in death. I understand that the physician treated the patient for several days for the mumps, when the entire difficulty arose from the teeth. I think it is frequently the case that a dentist could, in a very few moments, explain matters and remedy the difficulty where a physician does not know in what direction to look for the trouble. I hope the time will soon come when physicians and dentists will understand each other better, and neither try to treat cases which they do not understand.

DR. BENEDICT.—This calls to mind a circumstance which I knew of when I was studying in the office of my perceptor, at Mount Vernon, Ohio. A lady came into the office one day and stated that she had made up her mind to go east, in accordance with the recommendation of her physician, and that she was going to have her teeth treated, or fixed up, as she said, before she went. She was in ill health, and her physician had recommended her to spend the summer at the sea shore. Before she left the office finally we extracted nine teeth, the roots of which were too far gone to be saved. My preceptor inquired what medicine she was taking. She said her physician had told her it was not necessary for her to take anything excepting a blue pill. He told her he thought she had better abandon that. It proved that the whole difficulty came from the teeth, and in two weeks from the time of the removal of those teeth she was able to do a great deal of work about her house, abandoned her trip, and in less than a month reported that she was as well as she ever had been.

Dr. Barrett.—You will pardon me if I run counter to the feeling of a good many of the members of this society, to which I have so recently had the honor to be elected a member. In the paper which has just been read I find the opening statement that "The Michigan Dental Association, in its code of ethics, declares dentistry to be a specialty of medicine," etc. It is upon that statement that I wish to speak. Dentistry is not a specialty of medicine, and can only be made so in one way. There are three great professions that have existed since man had legal rights to conserve—since he had ills of body, and since he began to concern himself about a possible hereafter. The three professions of law, medicine and divinity have existed almost since the beginning of social time, and are the only three great professions that there are. The profession of letters is an outgrowth, the growth of a later day, and is not considered a profession in the strictest sense of the term. No man can be admitted to either of these three professions except in a regular way. No man can practice law without an examination by a competent board which, through a legal enactment, shall permit him to practice law in a legal way. No man is admitted to the pulpit, or allowed to become a teacher in theology, until he has gone through a regular course of study and been regularly admitted to the profession, and through some church organization. No man is permitted to practice medicine—at least no man is considered a member of the profession of medicine unless he comes in at the one door. Anyone who attempts to climb up any other way is a thief and a robber. A man cannot practice medicine legitimately until he becomes a medical man, and there is only one way in which he can do that, which is by obtaining a reputable medical diploma. We cannot call dentistry a specialty of medicine, as it is at present practiced. A shoemaker might as consistently claim to be practising a specialty of medicine as the average dentist. The dentist studies the anatomy of a certain portion of the body, the head, and the shoemaker the anatomy of a certain other portion of the body, the foot. The one is no more a medical man than the other, unless he becomes so in the regular way. I am not speaking now of the amount of knowledge which a man may possess, but I am speaking of the propriety of calling a man a specialist in a profession of which he is not a member. One cannot practice a specialty in medicine until he becomes a member of the medical profession. The opthalmologist is admitted to the medical profession only after he obtains his degree of M. D. The same is true of the gynecologist, the dermatologist, the otologist, or any other specialist in the medical profession. We complain sometimes that medicine does not acknowledge us. That is true, and it can acknowledge no one who is not an M. D. without stultifying itself from A. to Z. I will acknowledge that when I commenced dentistry I came into it by the back door. I was not one of the favored ones, and did not have the opportunities more lucky ones had of going through a college course. I had to work my way along, and go through college when I could. By making the best of the opportunities which I possessed, I finally did go through college and graduated an M. D. If I had known when I began the height of the mountain that stood before me I never would have attempted to climb it, because it is no trifling thing. The labor which I performed in those years has resulted in permanent injury to me. I shall never recover my digestive functions as they were before. When I became more familiar with medicine, and entered a medical college, I began to understand why it was that the profession could not consistently recognize those who are outside of it. I saw the absurdity of the claim made upon the profession. I then learned, what I now fully realize, that there is no other way by which a man has a right to claim to belong to the profession except to obtain his degree of M. D. in the regular way. When he has done that he may practice opthalmology, otology or dermatology, or any of the specialties. Under such circumstances, having done this, a man has no trouble in being recognized as a member of the profession—there is no obstacle in his way; but if a man, I do not care who he is, claims to be practising a specialty in medicine, without a medical degree, it is the height of absurdity. The most learned men living—like Huxley, Tyndall and Darwin—without their degree of M. D. or M. R. C. S., could not be considered medical men. The most learned D. D. in the world, though he be a man who has studied the most deeply, a man who has gone into metaphysics more thoroughly than anyone else, has no right to claim the title M. D. or to be a member of the profession. The most learned lawyer of the country, the Chief Justice of the United States, has no more claim to be considered a member of the medical profession than anyone else outside of it. A man might claim, with equal propriety, to be a member of the legal profession, and to be practising a specialty in it, because there is a legal side in medicine. It would be just as consistent to claim to be practising a specialty of law or a specialty of theology. The title D. D. S. has no more to do with medicine than LL. D. If a man is going to practice a specialty in medicine he must practice upon a higher plane than the man who practices it generally. I think the degree of D. D. S. is misleading. It is entirely separate and different from M. D. I know very well that this is unpalatable food for those who have earned the degree of D. D. S., but that does not lesson its truth. The

D. D. S. is required to study the anatomy of the head, but, as I said before, he studies it no more honestly than the scientific shoemaker studies the anatomy of the foot.

We must look this subject square in the face, and adopt one of two courses. If we are to practice a specialty in medicine, then we must first acquire the degree of M.D. This is one course, For my own part, however, I believe dentistry is strong enough to stand alone. There are certain advantages which might be gained by making a dental student first go through a course of medicine. But we must either become members of a medical profession or cease to claim to be. When we understand this matter thoroughly, there will be no more carping at our medical colleges. We know that we often hear such expressions as those which I find in this paper that, "The Michigan Dental Association declares dentistry to be a specialty of medicine," I think this is not only untrue, but something more—it is unwise. If a man is going to practice a specialty, he must prepare himself for it in a proper way. As far as I am concerned, I think dentistry has the right and the ability to stand independent from medicine. Shall it do this, or shall it go into the profession of medicine by the path which leads directly through the medical college? That is the question which the dental profession has to solve to-day.

Dr. Watling.—The gentleman is laboring under a misapprehension in regard to the course of study pursued in some dental schools. If he had attended the course and received the degree of D. D. S. from some dental schools, I imagine he would have had as thorough a knowledge of medicine as most medical students get. When he says the dental student is only required to dissect the head, and to receive a little smattering of a knowledge of medicine, he makes an assertion which I know is not true. I say our dental students are required to do the same dissecting as medical students, and are required to attend the same course of medicine very nearly. They receive the same instruction in chemistry as medical students do. The difference is the student who receives the degree of D. D. S. is certified to be a dentist, or to have gone through with the studies required to complete a course in dentistry, and the M. D. practices medicine. Dr. Barrett has taken the degree of M. D., and is practising a specialty in medicine. Does he operate any differently from what I do; does he fill teeth any better than I do, or use any more scientific agencies than I do? I doubt it. Is he any more successful in the treatment of diseased conditions? I doubt it. Yet he comes up and says we are no more practising medicine than a man who is making shoes; that the shoemaker is required to study the anatomy of the human body in order to make shoes successfully, and that he studies it as much as the dentist ordinarily does. I do not subscribe to any assertion of that kind. I think there is a great deal of unnecessary talk about degrees. It is a well known fact that many of our graduates attend a few lectures in a medical school, and receive the degree of M.D. Then they hawk it about as the first and most prominent thing, making it conspicuous on their sign as Dr. So-and-So, M.D., and then adding after it their degree of D. D. S. I have known of cases where, after perhaps two months of lectures in a medical school, dentists have received the degree of M. D. I know that is the case in Philadelphia. I know when Dr. Barrett asserts that dental students, as a rule, are only required to dissect a little of the head or to know a little of the anatomy of the head, he shows he is not familar with the course of study in some of the dental schools of this country.

Dr. Barrett—I did not say so. I said, as a rule, practitioners only do know that. I said nothing about the requirements of dental schools. I spoke of dentistry as commonly practiced.

Dr. Watling—Perhaps if you had gone through a regular dental college you might have had just as thorough a knowledge of medicine as you now have.

Dr. Barrett—I think you misunderstand me. I did not

say that dental students may not have the knowledge. I expressly stated that the most learned men on earth have no right to be received into the profession of medicine unless they have gone through with a regular course of medicine. I said especially that Tyndall, Huxley and Darwin cannot be accepted as medical men unless they have their medical degree. I make no attack upon any college or upon any person. Let nobody understand that I am criticising the University of Michigan. It is too large for me to handle. If their curriculum in the dental college is no different from the curriculum of medicine, they are setting a good example; but does the gentleman mean to assert that the dental student is required to attend the lectures upon gynecology and the practice of medicine. This is not the case in any school that I know anything about.

Dr. Watling.—That is where you are mistaken.

Dr. Barrett.—I did not suppose that a knowledge of gynecology was necessary for the practice of dentistry, or so considered in any dental school on earth, but it is necessary for medicine. It is something that the dentist is not supposed to practice at all, but in medicine it is absolutely essential. As far as the attaining of the degree of M. D. is concerned, I have no doubt that in Philadelphia a dental degree is as cheap as a medical degree. That used to be the case. I do not know any medical college which could give the degree of M. D. consistently to a dental student after one term. I know we have dental colleges that consider themselves reputable who give their degrees on one course of lectures. The statement that Dr. Watling makes that there may be no difference in knowledge, or only a slight difference, does not cover the ground I took. In order to be a member of the medical profession, it is not sufficient that you possess the knowledge, but you must have the evidence of the knowledge. Who is to give that evidence? Who is to be judge? I might just as consistently claim that I have sufficient knowledge to stand up and preach the gospel. I know a great deal about the gospel, but still I don't claim to be qualified for that, and I have very serious doubts as to whether I would be allowed to do that. I think I know something about law, but I could not go into the courts and practice. It is not safe to judge men always by the estimate which they put upon themselves, and there must be some competent body in all the professions—not only competent, but unbiased—which shall pass upon the claims of every man who aspires to be considered a member of the profession. The only way in which we can judge of a man whom we do not know is to take the judgment of the faculty and board of directors of a medical college.

I am not certain but dentistry is fully capable of standing alone, and making no claims or attempts in the direction of being considered a branch of medicine. I am not speaking of any one dentist in particular, or attacking any institution of learning. I am talking general principles, and I say, as a general principle, a man cannot become a member of the medical profession, or practice as a specialist in that profession, until he has obtained a degree in it in a legitimate manner. When he has obtained it, it is simply a matter of taste as to how he shall use it.

Dr. Wilson.—The National Medical Association has, I think, recognized dentistry, for it has established a section on dentistry.

Dr. Barrett.—Does not that apply to medical men who are practising dentistry—that is, who are practising a specialty in medicine, or does it refer to dentistry alone?

Dr. Wilson.—The section on dentistry has been established.

Dr. Barrett.—On "Oral diseases?"

Dr. Wilson.—It simply reads, "Section on dentistry."

Dr. Brophy.—That is a fact.

Dr. Wilson.—It is requisite for admission that the applicant be possessed of a medical degree. It was suggested that the name be made "Section on dentology," but it was made simply, "Section on dentistry.' I am glad they require a medical degree. I think the public will gradually be educated up to the necessity of dentists possessing a medical degree. The public are not prepared at present to compensate us for the services which we would give, or to pay us the extra amount of money which we would want for the addititional time spent in preparation. A great many dentists are practising without any degree, but I think the time is coming when the course in dental colleges will include a thorough knowledge of medicine. I think the courses in our dental colleges at present are much superior to what they have been in the past. I think the progress is in the right direction. For my part I attended almost all the lectures on practice of medicine, all the lectures on gynecology, and most of the lectures in all the departments. I am much in favor of the medical degree, and hope that in the future it will in all cases precede the dental degree.

DR. BARRETT—While I was speaking I did not realize the fact that I was in the State where the Michigan University is found. If I had, it probably would not have made any difference. I have said it before in other societies, and have met with a good deal of opposition because I said it, that the best schools we have are those in which there are professors of dentistry in medical colleges, and I think that as the result of these, the time is coming when the separate segregated schools must go to the wall.

DR. DORRANCE—In the Michigan University the department of dentistry is added to the medical department.

DR. BARRETT—I know that. I am not entirely ignorant about the University of Michigan, therefore I say that the segregated individual schools will, in time, be so far surpassed by the schools in connection with dental colleges that there will be little occasion for their existence. I have always been sorry that all the old teachers in dental schools did not go and unite themselves with the medical schools. Some of them have done so, and I think it is a step in the right direction. Michigan University is something that the State may well be proud of. There is no school which stands ahead of it that I know of. That and Harvard are two schools whose diplomas are admitted and recognized across the water. It is not altogether because of what they teach in the school itself, but because they require some preliminary knowledge, something showing that the student will not disgrace his profession by his ignorance. I would be ashamed of a profession that would admit every cross-road dentist, every ordinary peripatetic tooth puller, and call him a medical man.

DR. TAFT—How many medical colleges in this country require a preliminary examination? Is there any that require a preliminary examination equal to that in the dental department of the University of Michigan?

DR. BARRETT—I know of none.

DR. SHATTUCK—There is one in Detroit.

DR. TAFT—I am glad to know it, and I hope more will follow the good example, but the great body of the medical colleges makes no attempt in that direction. In most of the medical colleges anyone can enter, even though he cannot write his own name intelligibly or read a sentence of his mother tongue correctly. It is an unfortunate fact that those institutions which are dependent upon the support of the fees of the student, usually manage in some way to carry their students through. It is very seldom that students are dismissed from these institutions, no matter how great the provocation. So far as the endorsement of a diploma is concerned, I wish to say this: we find men in the profession who are a disgrace to it, and a disgrace to the community in every sense of the word. Let us take broad views on this subject of professional education and culture, and not conclude that the dental profession has all the incompetents and all the quacks, and that therefore we need to become members of the medical profession for our own protection.

DR. BARRETT—No one claims all that. All we claim is that their short comings don't excuse ours.

DR. TAFT—That is true, but let us put the responsibility

where it belongs, and let us not by implication say that everyone else is all right, and we all wrong; that because students may receive the sanction and endorsement of a medical faculty they are par excellence. A man who is worthy should receive the credit for all the attainments he has, even though he has not the sanction or endorsement of anybody. That is the position I take in regard to the matter. These endorsements are good so far as they go, but they are fearfully abused everywhere.

DR. BARRETT—I quite agree with Professor Taft in all that he has said, but this question arises whenever we discuss this subject: who is to judge of a man's attainments—who is to be the authority to decide? There are a great many unworthy men in all professions, but that does not dispose of the fact that some one must have the authority to decide who can and who cannot belong to a profession. A man may have all the qualifications, but without he is regularly admitted to the medical profession he has not the legal right to practice it. When some recognized organization, some authority on the subject gives him a diploma and certifies that he is qualified to practice medicine, it makes him a member of the medical profession in a legal way.

DR. TALBOT—Would it not have been better for the profession if the degree of D. D. S. had never been known? Would not the dental profession to-day have a better standing; would it not be looked upon by the community at large as being more proficient; would we not have a better standing as a profession if the degree of dental surgery had never been established, and if all dentists obtained their degree through medical colleges, as other physicians do?

DR. TAFT—I don't know whether it would have been better or not. I do not believe, under the circumstances, it would have been better if the degree of D. D. S. had never been created or known. I think that has been one of the great instrumentalities of elevating the profession. The medical colleges closed their doors agains us, we had no access to them,

Years ago we applied to the medical colleges for the establishment of chairs of dentistry, and the doors were closed against us. So the only way to get special education in this way was through an institution specially provided for it.

Dr. Barrett—That was one of the mistakes which medicine has made.

Dr. Taft—We ought not to be held accountable for that. I think if no dental colleges had been established, the dental profession would have remained in a low estate. It would not have been developed as it has been developed to-day. Had it not been for these schools the medicial colleges would have been closed to us to-day as they were then. The organization of dental colleges has been a very important influence in the creation of our literature. Associations have been established as the result of these schools, and a unity of feeling has resulted from them. So all the work that has been done for the elevation of dentistry, has been influenced, to a very great extent, by the special colleges which have been organized and by the work which they have done. Notwithstanding the fact that the day of their great usefulness may have passed away, we should remember them for the good they have done before. To-day the doors of the medical colleges are thrown open and the dentist is invited to come in. They now recognize us as an important branch or specialty of medicine. I think we would not have been anywhere near where we are to-day if these schools had never existed.

Dr. Talbot—What is our relation to the masses of people at large, as a separate profession? I would like to hear you speak upon that. Do our patients think as much of us, and do they heed what we say; do they recognize us as professional men, and do they regard our teachings as much as they would if it was generally understood that the path to success in dentistry lay through a regular medical education? Do they look upon us professionally with as much respect as they do upon the medical profession.

DR. TAFT—In some respects far more. In a community, an intelligent dentist is more highly esteemed than any man who is simply a physician can be in this particular direction. Medical men make some of the most egregious blunders in reference to diseases of the mouth, and when an intelligent person comes to compare them with able dental practioners, how do you suppose the dentist is esteemed? Is he not esteemed many times far above the physician in that particu lar direction? He will be found to be held at his true value, if not indeed far higher than he ought to be. How is it when you send a patient to a physician for the treatment of parts connected with the teeth and mouth, and the physician says, "I don't know anything about this. Dr. Talbot knows more about it than I do," and the patient comes back to you; under those circumstances how do you suppose the physician is estimated, as compared with the dentist. I have had that occur time and time again in my own practice, where patients have gone to consult a physician about affections of the mouth. In several instances I have sent patients to professors of medical colleges, and they have been returned without examination, the physician saying, in two instances at least, that he knew nothing about the case, and that they had better come back to me. How much better do you suppose the patient would esteem the dentist than the physician? Most assuredly, if he is a person of any judgment at all, the dentist will occupy a proper position in his estimation. There is no difficulty in making patients understand the ability of the dentist to treat cases of this kind.

DR. BARKER—All institutions are the result of a necessity. If there had been no necessity for the dental college, there never would have been one. It seems to me the dental college was established for a very good purpose. You may tell us it is all nonsense to have separate dental colleges, but it seems to me, nevertheless, that they would not have existed had there been no good cause for them.

Dr. Brophy—Dr. Taft has evidently practiced dentistry in a location where dentists are more highly respected than they are generally throughout our country.

Dr. Barrett—They have reason to respect them more perhaps.

Dr. Brophy—That is what I desired to say. He is not familiar with their habits so much as others who have lived further in the interior. It was only this week that I knew of a case, part of the history of which I will give you. A patient was consulting a dentist in regard to a disease of the teeth. An abcess formed which was not successfully treated, and it led on to necrosis. As soon as necrosis was discovered the dentist declared that it had gone beyond his reach, and that he had not the ability to treat anything beyond the tooth itself. The patient was therefore directed to a surgeon. Finally a portion of the bone was removed. Such cases do not leave a very good impression upon the mind of the patient or of the people of the city in which the patient resides, who were largely familiar with the case, owing to its notoriety. I say it is all wrong. Had that man known the principles of medicine and surgery he would not have humiliated himself by saying, "I am not able to go beyond the disease of the tooth itself." Cases like that occur too frequently. In Cincinnati, Detroit and Chicago, as well as other large cities, dentists do treat these diseases successfully, but this is not always so in the interior. There are fifty million people in this country, and only a few of them are fortunate enough to secure the services of the most skilled members of the profession. What do you suppose is the opinion that fifty million of people have of the dental profession to-day in regard to their scientific attainments in the treatment of disease?

Dr. Taft—What was the estimate in which this professor of a medical college was held by the patient when he returned him to me, saying he knew nothing of the affection under which the patient was suffering.

Dr. Brophy—I think the professor must have failed to state the case exactly as it was. He did know something about it. If he was a professor in a college he knew the principles governing the treatment of disease. If there was inflammation or suppuration, he knew what the remedies were to overcome them. There is no doubt about that. I think he had such confidence in Professor Taft's ability to treat the disease, that he was perfectly willing to leave the case to his care. Perhaps he had not the disposition to treat it, and therefore said, "I know nothing about it, go back to the professor."

Dr Taft—That is a very sugary way to get out of it.

Dr. Brophy—As to the relation of dentistry to medicine, I have this to say: Dentistry is or ought to be a branch of the great medical tree. I consider it just as much so as dermatology. What dermatologist to-day would be esteemed a medical man if schools were established for the object of giving instruction in that department alone. What would be thought of a school where dermatology alone should be taught? The same thing applies to gynecology, opthalmology and other parts of medicine. The man who would be a dermatologist, attends the lectures in all the parts of medicine and surgery. When he graduates he has a knowledge, not only of his specialty, but of the other departments of medicine, and the whole subject to which it is allied. when the same course is taken by dental students they will deserve to be called medical men. The only way in which we may become medical men, as Dr. Barrett has truly said, is through the medical institutions of our country. I do not say these institutions are all just exactly what they should be, but they are the best means of receiving an education for the treatment of diseases. When the time comes that these institutions will have professors who make the diseases of the teeth a specialty, and when the treatment of the teeth is only a part of the whole general course, the highest efficiency will be attained. Doctors will then be able to detect disease and refer patients who come to them to those best competent to treat them. It seems to me that this question is so clear it does not require very much argument. I have often said that when the time comes that dentistry is included in the curriculum of medical studies, and all medical men have the advantages of study in regard to the pathology of the teeth, they will do more good than all the dentists combined in assuaging or preventing diseases peculiar to the oral cavity, and we will hear no more of this talk about surgeons or physicians being ignorant in regard to the management of the oral cavity. They will be able to direct their patients to those who are competent to treat them.

DR. TALBOT—I hardly agree with all the remarks of Professor Taft. He says that a man is taken for what he is worth. I think that is not true in every case. If he will look at his own institution he will see that is not altogether true. I look upon the institution at Ann Arbor as the best of its kind in the country. He knows, and so do the other professors of the institution, that we in Chicago have made it a point to transfer our students from the east to that institution, knowing that it is progressive and that it is far in advance of any other in the country. We must all admit that. Dr. Taft says we are taken for what we are worth, but he must admit that while a young man who attends college and spends two or three years in the institution in which he is teaching, that young man is pretty well qualified if he has given attention to his lectures, to practice general medicine, yet this and other institutions confer upon each and every dental student an inferior degree. When a dental student attends the lectures, which are specified in the course, in the institution at Ann Arbor, and which include a great deal of instruction in the general practice of medicine, so much as to qualify him very well in this particular, he does not receive the degree to which he is entitled. He receives an inferior degree. I think the professor will admit that with a little extra study, a month or two perhaps, in some special branches, the dental student who has taken a course in the

University of Michigan is qualified to receive a medical degree. I think it is a matter of regret that when this result has been so nearly attained, anyone should be satisfied with the dental degree simply instead of going on and obtaining the full medical degree.

DR. HUNTER—I am opposed to calling dentistry a specialty of medicine. Of course there is no objection to a dentist's having a knowledge of as many branches of science as he is capable of attending to; but dentistry means just that. It means the treating of the diseases of the mouth, and that is our practice. We might as well call dentistry a specialty of mathematics, of mechanics or of minerology, because the dentist is supposed to have a knowledge of some of those sciences. It would be as appropriate to call it this as to call it a specialty of medicine. I am in favor of having every profession stand upon its own responsibility and its own merits. I am not in favor of begging from any profession as a profession. I am in favor of raising the dignity of our own profession by giving superior advantages and proper application to its study, selecting the right students, giving them the proper instruction so that they may be more skilled than even the best of us to-day. We are entitled to a place of our own and we can have it if we only stand upon it and build upon it, not begging from some one else.

DR. SHATTUCK—I think if Dr. Barrett and Dr. Hunter had attended a course in the University of Michigan, attended the lectures on gynecology or obstetrics, lectures on the practice of medicine and surgery, the same as the medical students attend there, either of them would have been willing to admit that dentistry is a specialty of medicine. I think it would have been perfectly plain to them. We should judge our profession by the best men in it, just as the legal profession is judged. We should think of it and judge of it as practiced by scientific men, men who have been educated for it, not by those who pick it up.

DR. BARRETT—According to your claim the students at the University of Michigan go through the same course as the medical students. If that is true, then why are they not given the medical degree?

DR. SHATTUCK—Simply because they have never entered their names for a medical degree.

DR. BARRETT—Could they get it?

DR. SHATTUCK—They could by studying longer.

DR. BARRETT—That bags the whole question.

DR. SHATTUCK—I think it is perfectly plain that such men are practicing dentistry as a specialty of medicine. I do not think that is so of all students, but I think it is so far as the graduates of the dental department of the University of Michigan are concerned.

DR. DORRANCE—I know of one case which occurred where a gentleman took a degree in medicine after he had attended the lectures in the dental department, and received the full degree of M. D. before he received his dental degree. I do not know what his previous attainments were.

DR. BARRETT—Had he never attended any lectures before?

DR. DORRANCE—I do not know.

DR. BARRETT—If he had gone through a course somewhere else that would change the situation.

DR. CLWSAON—I will take Dr. Barrett at his own statement, He graduated in medicine and in dentistry I believe, and now says his health is injured by his having so done. Is not that the case with the American people generally? Are they not trying to do too much? I believe if we are to practice dentistry we ought to bring in everything that helps to make good practitioners, but I think we are asking a little too much and trying to do too much in a limited time. We break down too early from that very fact. I think it is all wrong to attempt to do so much in so short a time.

DR. ALPORT—My views upon this subject are so well understood that it is hardly worth while for me to say much in regard to it. In my judgment dentistry as it is practiced at the present time, that is to say if we reckon it as a profession by itself, and as it should be practiced rather than as it is practiced, is so extended that we can hardly perfect ourselves in it in any dental college or anywhere else in the time that is now allotted to it. The only correct way to properly learn the practice of dentistry as we practice on the other organs or relieve and heal disease, is to go through the same curriculum that the students in other departments of medicine have to go through. Then, if they desire to engage in the practice of a specialty and call it a specialty in medicine, they are enabled to do it. If they wish to practice in the mechanical department of dentistry, let them enter it as a distinct calling and follow it as such. I do not think the time is sufficient for any considerable number of men to learn what we call dentistry to-day, and practice in both departments correctly, or even acceptably to the people. If we are going to become physicians, as anyone ought who intends to practice the curing of any disease, there is but one way to qualify ourselves for it.

Dr. Dorrance—In my opinion there is no one man who is able to practice medicine in all its branches. There was a time when there were no medical colleges. We have them now, not only for the purpose of instruction, but also for the purpose of controlling the profession. Dentistry has very rapidly passed through about the same stages that medicine once passed through. A few years ago a dentist was of little more consequence than a barber. He was not a medical man in any sense of the word. The medical man on the other hand did not enter into the subject of the treatment of diseases of the mouth as he did into gynecology and other diseases of the body. To my mind dentistry, gynecology, dermatology or any other ology connected with the study of medicine are not capable of being separated or graded in importance. There is no apparent distinction between them in importance. One is as of much consequence as the other, but to be thoroughly perfected in the practice of any one of these branches requires special study and fitness, and no man can fit himself for any of these specialties in a short time. In dentistry, particularly, there is no one man in five hundred who is able to thoroughly practice both branches. He must possess extraordinary requirements to succeed as a practitioner in the treatment of diseases of the mouth, and also in mechanical dentistry. He may have a fair medical education, as it is called, and I consider this almost indispensable to the highest success in the treatment of diseases of the mouth, but he will be an exceptional man if he can practice both branches successfully. I consider dentistry as much a specialty of medicine as any other specialty of medicine can be. It is entitled to be recognized as such. We very well know that the best men in the dental profession are looked up to by the best men in the medical profession for their skill in the treatment of diseases of the mouth. The people recognize us; they recognize a man for what he is worth. The lights in the profession are recognized and trusted by the people. Those who are not worth recognizing should not be recognized and usually are not. In the case cited by Dr. Brophy, who was it that could not treat the teeth? Was it Dr. Brophy or Dr. Barrett or Dr. Taft? Not by any means. It was some one who did not know the first principles of his profession.

DR. BROPHY—He was a graduate of a dental college

DR. DORRANCE—He did not know what he was about at all events. This is a matter which must be considered in its proper light, and it is high time we did so. We cannot change it so far as some of us individually are concerned, but we must look out for those who are to follow. My belief is that a dentist's education should be based upon a general medical education. Crowding all the necessary instruction into too short a space of time is ill advised. A man cannot learn everything in a day. He must take time to fit himself for his chosen work. I believe that a youth who has any idea of practicing dentistry should be qualified first by a literary course, a medical course, and for his special dental work. In reference to the statement made as to the length of time required in order to graduate in the medical department, I wish to say that I believe a dental student who has been taking a course of lectures in the dental department of the University of Michigan cannot graduate an M. D. with any additional two months study.

DR. TALBOT—Of course I do not know whether it would take two months or a year, but I say a young man would do better to take the extra amount of time and obtain the degree of M. D. It would be better to take even two years more if necessary.

DR. DORRANCE—I agree with you as to that. The point of difference is simply as to the matter of time. I think the time spent in obtaining a medical degree is well spent, but it requires study and manipulation which cannot be obtained in any short period of time.

DR. BROWN—Speaking about this matter of sending a patient to a physician, in cases where you do not feel like taking the responsibility, I hardly know how we are going to get around it. Only a few months ago I had a patient come to my office with a malignant tumor of the inferior maxillary, extending to the second bicuspid. The other molars were gone. She had once submitted to an operation, and as she supposed, had a tumor removed, but when she came to me it was very large and seemed to affect the whole jaw. I did not feel like undertaking the amputation of the jaw, and doubt whether there is anyone here present who would. I advised my patient to go to Dr. McLean at Ann Arbor, which she did. The operation was successfully performed. If there are any members of this Association who would have performed that operation, I would like to know it, because in cases of this kind I would rather confer with men in the dental profession than in the medical profession.

DR. DORRANCE—I think Dr. Brown did well, but I say that the time is coming when a dental practitioner must necessarily do this sort of work and should be fitted for it. It is only recently that surgeons have recognized that there is something in reference to the human system which they did not know about. It is only recently they have found out that tumors may originate from conditions directly connected with the dental organs, or at least recognized that fact sufficiently to enable them to serve their patients more intelligently.

Dr. Allport—It is well known, or at least should be, that whoever operates about the mouth, and is familiar with those parts can perform more skillful operations than any surgeon in the world; the same as a man accustomed to operate about the eye can perform operations of that particular character better than any ordinary surgeon. I would like to ask the gentlemen who have just spoken if they had received a regular medical education and been thoroughly informed in the pathology of that class of diseases, if they had been educated in the principles of surgery, had attended clinics in surgery, in other words if they had received a full medical training beside their dental education, would they not have been more competent to have performed the operation which one of them has mentioned than any surgeon could be?

Dr. Parker—Sometimes a definition will help us. I would like to ask the doctor what he means by the word medicine in the present instance. Does he mean the art curative.

Dr. Barrett—I am speaking of medicine in the sense in which we all use it, as an incorporated profession which is bound by certain laws, the members of which are unequal in knowledge, some of whom are far more skilled than others, but all having gone through a certain curriculum of study, received a medical diploma and regularly received into the medical profession. I am not speaking of medicines nor their curative properties, but of medicine as a profession; men who have a right to belong to it, and who are in the line of demarkation, who have entered the gate which admits them to fellowship as medical men.

Dr. Parker—Does not all that mean simply that they have a right to practice the art curative—the ethical right?

Dr. Barrett—Yes, sir. It seems to me that medicine means the curative art, just as law or theology may be briefly defined according to their meaning. If that is so any man who practices any curative art, practices a part of medicine. It may be a specialty, as all parts are specialties, but I cannot see how you can dodge the conclusion that any man who practices any part is practicing the art of medicine, whether he is a dentist or a chiropodist.

Dr. Barrett—But is he practicing in the medical profession?

Dr. Parker—If you narrow it down to those who have diplomas that is a different thing, but if one is practicing the art curative you cannot dodge the conclusion that he is practicing a specialty of medicine.

Dr. Brophy—How would you define dentistry?

Dr. Barrett—I would define it as the practice of curing diseases of the teeth.

Dr. Parker—If dentistry is the curing of the teeth, and the teeth are a part of the body, I do not see how you can dodge the conclusion that dentistry is a part of medicine.

Br. Brophy—I expected to hear Dr. Barrett say a great deal more when asked to define dentistry. I shall not attempt to define it, but I desire to make a statement in regard to the legal aspect of this whole thing. As a dentist is a graduate of a dental college, and has obtained the degree of D. D. S., he ought to be legally authorized, if he is practicing medicine, to prescribe remedies. We know that he is not, at least in Illinois. Before one has a legal right to prescribe remedies, even in the treatment of diseases of the teeth, he must obtain a certificate from the State board of health. He is not legally qualified to prescribe remedies, no matter if he has the degree D. D. S. or any other degree, provided he has not been examined by the State board of health, or obtained a medical diploma. I think if we are specialists in medicine we ought to have the right to prescribe the remedies which are necessary in our own line.

DR. DORRANCE—That is a right which you should have.

DR. BROPHY—Dentists should have that right if qualified. As I say the law requires that a man who desires to prescribe shall either be a medical graduate, or pass an examination before the State board of health in all the departments of medicine.

DR. SHATTUCK—It seems to me if one gets a diploma, authorizing him to prescribe for diseases of the mouth, he ought to be allowed to prescribe for them. I think Dr. Barrett's idea is too closely drawn. Taking scientific dentistry, as it is practiced to-day, I think it is a part of medicine.

DR. BARRETT—I hope no one will understand me as undervaluing dentistry. I am not speaking about the qualifications of a dentist at all. I am sorry to hear Dr. Talbot speak of the degree of D. D. S. as an inferior degree. You cannot draw any distinction between M. D. and D. D. as to which superior or inferior, and the same thing applies to the dental degree. I was simply saying that a man as a dentist is not necessarily a member of the medical profession, and that he cannot be unless he has been admitted to the profession in the regular way. For my part I think dentists are able to take care of themselves, and should not be creeping into medicine until they come in at the regular door.

DR. DORRANCE—We do not want to.

DR. BARRETT—What is the statement in the code of ethics of the Michigan Dental Association for, then?

DR. DORRANCE—I do not know, I did not put it there.

DR. BARRETT—It is not fair or truthful to make a claim of that kind until we come in the regular way. Here we have the statement, "The Michigan State Dental Association in its code of ethics declares dentistry to be a specialty in medical science."

DR. DORRANCE—Who has said anything about it being a specialty in the medical profession?

DR. BARRETT—I understand the term "medical science" to mean the medical profession.

DR. DORRANCE—Not necessarily. The statement is not that the dental profession is a specialty of medicine, but it says dentistry. It does not make the distinction between the profession of dentistry and the profession of medicine. It makes the claim that dentistry is a specialty of medical science.

DR. BARRETT—I am taking the ordinary, common acceptation of the term. Perhaps strictly speaking I am not correct. *Haec fabula docet.* Moral: We cannot any of us know too much.

DR. TALBOT—I would like to define my position in regard to my use of the expression "inferior degree." I meant to say that it was an inferior degree, as looked upon by the masses of the people. Most of our patients do not know what the degree of D. D. S. means, while they do know what M. D. means.

DR. WATLING—They do not know what M. D. means; they do not understand it.

DR. DORRANCE—I doubt not if you and Dr. Talbot keep on practicing they will know what D. D. S. means.

DR. MILLER—I would like to ask my friend from Illinois, if a dentist is not legally allowed to prescribe for diseases of the teeth, who is? Is the M. D. allowed to, who knows but little about the teeth.

DR. BROPHY—What I undertook to say was that a dentist had no right to write a prescription. He can use remedies in his own office, but he has no legal right to write a prescription for the treatment of diseases which require constitutional treatment, such as every intelligent dentist must treat.

DR. CLAWSON—It seems to me the Illinois law is rather absurd, it does not give the dentist a chance to do what he ought to in a great many cases.

DR. HARLAN—I think there is a little misapprehension in reference to the law in Illionois. I helped pass that law, and I think we have as much the advantage of the medical profession as they have of us. A man who has the degree of M. D. cannot practice dentistry unless he obtains a certificate from the State board of dental examiners. I do not know what other D. D. S's. do, but I write prescriptions every day, and the drug stores fill them. As I understood it the degree of D. D. S. confers the right to prescribe for any diseases of the mouth.

Dr. Whiting—I have been opposed to all these medical laws. If I go back to my native town, where I learned dentistry forty years ago, and extract a tooth, I am liable to a fine of twenty-five dollars. That is because I have not a license to practice dentistry there. I think we have no business to pass such laws. It is all very well to say we want to drive out quacks. We drive out just as good men as we have in the profession.

Dr. Dorrance—No profession has ever desired a law to protect the profession. These laws are designed to protect the people against quackery. I do not think any member of any profession who is skilled has ever thought it necessary that he, personally, should be protected against quackery.

Adjourned to 2 P. M.

AFTERNOON SESSION.

THE MOUNTING OF ARTIFICIAL CROWNS ON NATURAL ROOTS.

Dr. Dorrance—There can be no question, I think, in the minds of those who are present, as to the utility of the root that frequently comes to us with the crown gone. Even a diseased root, if the disease has not progressed too far, may be made exceedingly useful and should not be extracted, but some method adopted to preserve it. The root will not only give support to something that will enable the individual possessing it to masticate to better advantage on account of the increased surface, but it also assists in the retention of the other teeth in their position, and in the retention of the process preventing absorption and the consequent sinking of the muscles of the face and the contraction of the jaw. There is another reason still, and that is that people decidedly object to wearing artificial plates, putting it off as long as they can. Therefore some means of saving these roots in as good condition as possible should be pursued. Some of these methods have been in use a great many years. I do not know how many years ago the root was first used in some shape as a support to an artificial crown. I know that within the last few years quite a number of improved methods have been presented to us, which are far superior to the simple pivoting of the artificial crown, without protection to the root. Within the last few years we have been enabled to place crowns upon roots with the roots fully protected against any further loss of substance, and against the action of the secretions of the mouth or other agencies which would tend to destroy them. I will glance over a few of these methods hastily. For instance, a root in very bad condition, very much wasted may many times be saved in a very simple manner by the construction of a platinum band or ferule, and placing it upon the root, building up a crown thereon with amalgam. This method will save some roots that cannot support a crown with a pivot. We have, we will say, the root of a lower bicuspid, which is in a healthy condition, so far as the support of it is concerned. It is below the gum and may indeed be split through the weakness which has followed the loss of so much of its substance. Having filled the root with amalgam, a very simple and inexpensive way, I will explain the method of forming the ferule, which I consider the most expedient. There are a number of ways, but this is the simplest one. Dr Taft, I believe, originated it, at least he suggested it to me. I first take a strip of platinum sufficiently long to enable me to more than surround the root and place it upon the root. Then with the pliers I draw the ends together, getting a tight fit around the root. I then solder the ends together, letting them lap slightly. In this way I get a ferule fitting the root. That can be used in what is called the Richmond crown. It is really a very simple method. Of course the roots should be in a healthy condition and thoroughly cleansed. Pains should always be taken to prepare the root, so that in case of accident you may be able to remove whatever supports you may have placed in position. The method of putting into a root a support or pivot in such a manner that it is impossible to remove it, or very difficult to remove it is not a good one. In attempting to drill out the material which you have put in you will find that if these barbed pivots, which cannot be readily withdrawn have been used, the drill will be run out on one side or the other through the tooth, or into the structure of the tooth, for there is so much of the substance of the tooth gone that the resisting power of what is left is very slight.

Another method is to take a plate tooth and put a platinum cap on it. The method is very simple, and I do not know who to credit it to.

DR. HARROUN—An Italian dentist by the name of Maggiola used it in 1807.

DR. DORRANCE—Taking the platinum cap and putting it on the root a hole is made through it, entering the canal. The plate tooth is thus fastened on. The platinum cap is simply intended as a protection to save the root from further loss. A pin of any suitable material, gold, platinum or steel may be used. I have seen a steel pin used on a tooth which was probably inserted some forty years ago. The pin was inserted without any protection into the root, and worn for a long time. In this method this pin, we will say, crowded down into the root, no attempt being made to restore the form of the tooth, but simply allowing the tooth, with its backing of gold, to act as a support to the crown. There is no attempt made to fill out the shape of the tooth.

A MEMBER—Why not?

DR. DORRANCE—I am simply explaining a very easy operation. I am not saying what we might do, but what has been done. No doubt it might be done. Some other method may be pursued to better advantage, no doubt, in many cases, but I am giving you at a glance the methods which have been used, and are still used. This makes a very fair operation, rather crude it is true, but highly successful in many cases, teeth having often been preserved for a long period of years.

DR. HARROUN—That operation can be easily performed by putting platinum in the root instead of gold.

DR. DORRANCE—Yes, the restoration can be made with the same material; but what I call particular attention to is the protecting of the root with a platinum cap. I am illustrating that method only. Dr. Webb introduced the plan some years ago, in 1872 or '3 I think, of using a plate tooth in that way.

He ground away a plate tooth, and then placed a split ferule on the backing, so that it nearly closed around it, but leaving it so that it would spring a little. Having done that he slid the tooth, with its ferule, up on to the pin which was built into the root itself.

Another way, which is of particular use on the front teeth, and perhaps also in treating the posterior teeth, is this: after putting in a plastic filling, and making a tapering opening in the filling, making a pin with a screw thread, and fastening it into the tooth in that way. I have seen teeth which have been used for a long time after having been screwed in and they kept their place very well. Some means must be taken to protect the root, or in a few years it is wasted and gone.

Another method of holding the crown, the origin of which I do not know, but which I first used in 1871, was this: I put a tooth in place by fastening it to the teeth adjoining. A great many attempts have been made in the same direction, but in a good many instances the operation has been unsuccessful and resulted to the sorrow of those who tried it. I will tell you the reason why there have been so many failures. The attempt has been made in various ways to support a tooth where there was no root at all by completely and firmly attaching it to two other teeth. If this is done it will uniformly result in injury to the adjoining teeth. Something will happen. We know that the teeth have a motion which must be allowed them. The teeth are not firmly fixed in their sockets, but must be allowed to change their position slightly whenever they strike upon any firm substance, and in fact at all times during the process of mastication. I will try and reveal to you the secret of attaching teeth in such a way that no injury will result. The method is that of placing a backing upon the tooth and using either a transverse or longitudinal arrangement of pins, preferably the longitudinal, cutting out a section at the point indicated in my diagram, with the wheel, so as to leave a little space and introducing two gold lugs on either side of sufficient length, and with a bend in them which is allowed by the curve which I show you in the diagram. These gold lugs come out on either side. It is simply a matter of manipulation to put them in place. It is not necessary for me to tell those familiar with the work how to do that. I do not recommend making cavities in the teeth to do this. I believe in letting well enough alone. But supposing there are cavities in the adjoining teeth, say in the left central and right lateral teeth, these cavities may be freely filled, with this exception. Taking either one of these cavities, that in the left central for instance. In one or the other of these or both, you have a place cut or left in the filling which will receive one of the lugs. In one of them you must necessarily finish the filling after the tooth is put in. So the cavity is left unfinished, the other being filled. Then go on and insert the lug into the second one, and drop it back into the groove left for it. Then proceed to finish the filling. That leaves the tooth movable to a certain extent. The crown should fit nicely. During the operation the mouth should be protected with a thin rubber dam, the tooth adjusted in its place and then dried. If you follow this method of finishing the filling in one of the teeth after you have inserted the gold lug you will find it works well. If you build it into the filling after you have finished it it will not get the necessary motion. Where you have cavities in the adjoining teeth I think this a good method to pursue. I think the objections to it are no greater than those which apply with equal force to others which are less preferable.

Dr. Talbot—I believe in the insertion of artificial crowns upon the roots of natural teeth, and think it is one of the most interesting, as well as durable, operations which can be performed at the present day. I think we should try and perfect the process as much as possible. I do not think we have yet found perfection in it, although we have unquestionably made rapid advances. I have studied this subject considerably, but am not able to advance many original ideas. The crown that I believe to be of the greatest benefit to the patient, and the one that gives the dentist the most satisfaction is what is called the Richmond crown. This crown is now used in the west to a greater extent than in the east. The objection raised by our friends in the east is that the insertion of this crown irritates the gums and periosteum, causing them to slough and recede. I do not believe this, at least I do not think it objectionable to the extent that is claimed. While in San Francisco a couple of years ago, I took particular pains to hunt up a number of cases and saw a number that had been inserted upon natural roots, some six years ago and some ten years ago. These were in perfect condition at that time. Believing that the Richmond crown, as it it is called, is one of the greatest inventions of the profession, I tried to trace its history. I furnished an article for the Dental Cosmos, thinking I had found the originator of the crown, Dr. Biers of San Francisco, who took out a patent for it in 1862. Since I returned I have found that Dr. W. N. Morrison, of St. Louis, is the inventor of the crown. He inserted the first crown of this kind about three years previous to this time. Both Dr. Biers and Dr. Richmond improved on it very much. The main point in the success of this operation I believe to be the treatment and preparation of the root of the tooth, so that the crown will stand perfectly straight, so that it will be perpendicular, its support being in line from the edge of the root down to the alveolar process. This is accomplished by training the hand in the use of the excavator, and testing it by drawing it upward and downward in the tooth. Of course the roots must be first treated and filled before the operation can be performed, then select a piece of gold which should be rolled out to about 28 or 32 in thickness United States gauge, coin gold. Then bend it so that the edges touch, and put it down upon the root, between the root itself and the alveolar process. Then with round-nosed pliers bend the piece of gold and shape it to the root, bending it to as nearly the size of the root as you can by testing it. Then with the shears cut off the superfluous pieces of gold and you have the two edges coming together. The gold will fit accurately to the root of the tooth. It should then be secured by soldering. After this is done drive the gold band on to the root of the tooth till it reaches nearly or quite to the alveolar process. After you have accomplished this take a piece of wax and obtain the bite pressing it down on the gold band and to the teeth adjoining on either side. Cool it and remove the wax. Then remove the band. This can be done by running the excavator under the gum and pulling the band off. Insert the band into the wax and pour on the plaster. You then take the impression upside down. After you have taken this impression, obtain the impression of the teeth on the opposite side. You then have the condition of things which you find with the band driven on to the root and the teeth in the mouth. If the band should be a little longer than is necessary it should be trimmed. After this is completed flow the solder and you obtain the shape of the tooth. Finish it up nicely, dry the tooth, gum etc., thoroughly, and then force it on. In that way you have it just as you wish it. Remove it again, place in the cement. I generally use phosphate of zinc to fasten it on. If the operation has been accurately performed and the band fitted tight, I claim it makes the most durable crown we can put in the mouth. I think it is Dr. Richmond's plan, and I am unable to improve upon it. I have made one or two crowns, one of which I illustrated in the Dental Cosmos, where the root was decayed. I made a gold band in the same way that I have described, fitting it to the root of the tooth, then removing it, and soldering a piece of gold through the center, drilling a couple of holes through the band, and putting in a couple of screws, running them down into the root, then making a crown and fastening it on in the same manner represented in my first drawing. The difficulty with such an operation is that it is too expensive for the price a person would be likely to obtain for it.

Dr. Barrett—How do you fasten on your crown?

DR. TALBOT—With oxy-phosphate of zinc or some of the cements.

DR. BARRETT—Yes, but how do you fasten it on?

DR. TALBOT—I drive it down like the cover of a box.

DR. MOORE—How do you cut down the sides of the root to make them parallel, or nearly parallel?

DR. TALBOT—I take an instrument something like the shape of scalers, place it under the gum and work from the apex of the root up toward the crown.

DR. DORRANCE—I wish to say one word further relating to the methods that I have been talking about. I make this suggestion that you may very nicely accomplish the shaping of the crown by taking impressions of a half dozen different ones, of various sizes, in plaster, and striking them up. By a little practice a great deal can be accomplished in the way of gaining facility in shaping crowns.

You will find in filling the root, or in building the crown on it, you must necessarily provide some means of support to the crown besides the ferule, in a great many cases. In filling the apex of the root you will find the use of a little wire of lead will be very nice, dressing it down, so by constant trying you get it so it fills the cavity, and by taking means to ascertain the length of the canal, you may carry that up to the end of the canal, and pack it. It makes a very good filling for the apex of the root. Some prefer Hill's Stopping, others want gold. There are also a great many other materials. Some like cotton, and it is very good. I like lead as well as anything. I think a great deal of injury is done in driving ferules on to the roots of the teeth. There should be some care exercised in it. Some recommend lancing the gum about the root so as to make it less injurious, claiming that the application of the lance is less injurious than the tearing of the tissues.

DR. BARRETT—It has been objected that the ferule about the roots of the tooth will irritate the root and gum so much as to cause exfoliation. I have never found it so. I do not generally indulge in telling stories, or relating incidents, but I do wish to speak of one case. I put one of these crowns on two years ago, and since then the tooth has been broken, so I attempted to remove the crown, and I declare to you that I had more trouble to get it off than to get it on. I think if I had pulled it squarely off I would have taken the root with it. I had to grind the ferule off. I could not get it off in any other way, it was on so close. I put on a bicuspid tooth the same as I put on a central incisor or incisor-cuspid. In soldering on a tooth, I grind off a little from the corner, from the labial side sufficient to give room to flow in the solder. Now, the cylinder is fitted on just the same as in any other tooth.

I will attempt briefly to give my method of putting on crowns, hoping that I may give you as clear an idea as possible. A patient comes to me, for instance, with a lateral incisor broken off, or I find it so far gone that it cannot be saved. The first thing I do, if the nerve canal is in an irritable condition, if there is any soreness about the tooth, or it has not been previously filled or treated, is to treat the nerve canal till it is in a healthy condition. Then I fill the apex of the root. Then I grind it down level with the gum, or a little below the gum. I grind it down a little in the center with a round burr. The roots of the tooth have been filled a quarter or a third of the way up. I do not attempt to make any notches or any screw thread, or anything of that kind in the interior of the root. I enlarge the nerve canal so I can put a pin into it of sufficient size to hold the pivot. The next thing I do is to take some gold 30 or 32 thick, using a strip half an inch wide and wrap it around the end of the root. First, if I find the shape of the tooth falls away any, I make it as level and as even as I can. That is the second point. With my pliers I shape the gold as carefully as I can, fit it and burnish it till I get it down as close as I can. Then with a pair of nippers I wrap it around the tooth till one end strikes the other, mark it with an excavator at the point which I think is about right. It is only around the end of the root, but I mark it at the place which looks about right to me. If it goes on easily over the root, without spreading, it is a little too large, so I file away one of the ends a little and bring them together again. Finally I slip the gold over the end of the root till it spreads a little. I burnish it down till I get a good fit, bringing the ends together and soldering it. If I get it a little too tight I draw it out a little, making the edges of the lower side sharp. Now I try it on and see if it is all right. I put it over the end of the root, get my mallet and a piece of hickory wood and have them all ready. I do not say anything to the patient about this, because it is not an enjoyable part of the process to him. I put it in place, put my piece of hickory across it, and with the mallet I give two or three sharp blows, driving it up firmly until it is so fastened on the root that I am going to have a pull to get it off. Having got this in place, the next thing I do is to dress down the band until I have got it about the right length in the mouth. Then I go to work and put in the pin. I let it stick up a little. I use some material that will stand the heat. Platinum does very well, and gold is very good. I get a tooth of the right size and do the necessary grinding to give it the right shape. I grind it until it fits, or until I have got it just as I want it. The tooth is then laid one side and I prepare my modeling compound and take an impression. My girl uses a syringe with cold water, and throws water all around the tooth, cooling and cleansing it. I have my modeling compound pretty soft. The girl throws the water on it until she has chilled it so it is stiff and hard.

Now I have a perfect impression of the tooth with the pin in place. The next thing to do is to get off the band, which is no easy task if I have it swedged on as closely as it ought to be. Having this band taken off from the root, and having a sharp clear impression, it is an easy matter to fit on the tooth. A good deal depends upon getting a sharp, clear impression. I do not take any plaster cast, but use the modeling compound instead. Taking this impression in the modeling compound

I have not only the shape of the pin sticking up from the root, but the model of the teeth on each side. I next go to work and dress the pin down with the level of the rest. I next put my tooth in place on the model. I stick it fast with some wax. I have a perfect mental picture of it. Here I have a lateral incisor and a model of the teeth on each side of it, one on each side, and my impression of the root, with the edges of the band sticking up around it. So I can put my tooth in place where it belongs. I then flow in 18 carat gold till it is all solid. In my description I have left out one thing which has just come to my mind. It should have been done before. I refer to backing up of the tooth. I have some platinum rolled out as thin as I can get it, just like tissue paper. That is sufficient to back up the tooth with. I always back it up so the solder may flow on it. I am not particular whether it is a rubber tooth or not if I am satisfied it is a good one. Rubber teeth do not always stand the heat. I do not use the mouth blow-pipe, but use the Fletcher furnace blow-pipe. Putting my material on a piece of pumace stone. I heat the whole thing up until the solder flows nicely, keeping my blast going until the material runs easily. I use platinum sponge because it attracts the solder better. Platinum sponge is nothing more or less than platinum and gold. I have it so that zinc will run through it the same as water through a sponge, till it is a perfect solid mass. After it is cooled down I polish it up, and that is all there is to do, except to put it in place. I seldom try this on because I don't consider it necessary. I am perfectly satisfied it will go in place. There is no difficulty about that. In this stage of the process which I have described—the soldering, it is necessary to use a pretty high heat. When this is all finished up I dress the tooth a little more to make room for the cement. I allow a vent from the cavity, which I fill with oxy-chloride cement. I then put the crown in place, take my piece of hickory wood, place it on the tooth, giving two or three sharp blows, driving it to place until it is solid. Then the operation is done. Of course there are some things which must be taken into consideration all the time. You must see that your occlusion is going to be right, and that the tooth is not going to strike out of line. The pivot that I use has no barb or screw thread or anything of that kind. There is sufficient cement to make it fit tighter. I do not fill the root with cement, as a usual thing.

Dr. Dorrance—How would you do if the canal was very large?

Dr. Barrett—If the canal was large I would put cement in. If the tooth was decayed, so there was a great chamber in it, I would put in cement and might give a little shoulder to the cavity in the canal, so that the crown would be sure to stay, or would be a little more firm. I find though, that if the pivot is well driven home there is not the slightest liability to move, and if it is done well the crown is very firmly fixed, and there is no danger of its coming off under any ordinary circumstances. This operation I consider the most perfect piece of work in dentistry. I know of nothing so satisfactory as that. The root is perfectly protected, and the crown is so firm and solid that its possessor will masticate on it with all ease. I have put on a good many of these crowns which are so firm that I believe I could take hold of the crown and pull the root out.

Dr. Case—I have been very much pleased with the discussion so far, because I have put on a number of teeth in almost exactly the same way as Dr. Barrett, with the exception that in taking the impression, instead of taking the crown from its place after having it in place, I take the impression with it on, drawing the crown off from the root after the pin is fitted.

Dr. Barrett—You do not take an impression of the whole thing.

Dr. Case—Not on each side. This way was suggested to me some time ago by Dr. Dorrance.

Dr. Dorrance—I wish to impress, particularly, the necessity of the use of the thin platinum. When it is of the proper thickness you can shape it very easily, and in soldering, if you have no platinum sponge, you can use the gold foil just as well. I presume it is not generally known to the profession that there are ways of working metals much more simple than those taught in the books. Metal workers learn new things as well as other people. You can get at the platers' supply establishments a material which you will find very useful, called composition. It is a waxy compound of fine emery and crocus. You will find it of great service in some stages of the finishing. Apply the composition to the edge of the wheel with which you are polishing, and you will find that you can do much better work. I would like to call your attention again to the statement which I made that it will be better to use a screw thread pivot or pin where it is possible to do so. A short time ago I knew of a case where a man had received a blow from a ball which struck him in the mouth. He had a lateral incisor inserted in the way I speak of with a screw. The blow which he received bent the lateral incisor slightly. If the tooth had been fastened with a pin, it would probably have drawn out, and I would have the work to do over again. As it was the deflection was so slight I was able to bend it back again as it was, just before the accident.

Dr. Brophy—I desire to say that if the phosphate of zinc is used there need be no difficulty about removing the crown. If the crown be put on the way described by Dr. Barrett, Dr. Talbot and others, the cavity then being filled with phosphate of zinc, and the crown forced into position, and maintained in that way for a sufficient length of time, it will become quite hard. If at any time it becomes necessary to remove the ferule, it can be done very easily. Inserting the rubber dam upon the tooth pretty well up beneath the gum, take a hot air syringe and heat the tooth. The phosphate of zinc yields very readily to the influence of heat. It will become softened, and then with the forceps you may very easily remove the ferule. The tooth of course has been previously broken off.

Dr. Barrett—I wish to call attention to one or two points. With reference to the ease with which this operation can be performed. There are a good many who never have tried it, and to whom it seems, no doubt, quite difficult. Before I tried it I thought so myself. I did not succeed very well the first time or the second. A great deal depends upon having the materials in the right shape. The gold which is used should be rolled out to the proper degree of thinness. Coin gold will do very well. Platinum, when used, should also be very thin.

Dr. Dorrance—If the members of the Society wish to make a few experiments in this direction I will advise them to pursue the method spoken of by Dr. Talbot, I think. Take a few teeth which have been extracted from well formed crowns of different sizes, make some zinc dies, fasten the teeth in plaster so that they can be readily handled. Take some thin gold and make some crowns. You may leave them with the gold projecting a little. Strike up a few of these crowns and you will find the experiment a very interesting and advantageous one.

Dr. Barrett—About what thickness of gold would you recommend?

Dr. Dorrance—24 to 26.

Dr. Bean—I do not think sufficient stress has been given to the fact that it is necessary in mounting these crowns, and in putting in the cement, to leave a vent hole. I have seen cases where much irritation was occasioned by the soft cement being pressed up on the periosteum of the root. That could all be overcome by leaving a vent hole.

Dr. Parker—I wish to explain a method which I have been using a little in the mounting of these crowns. Instead of striking up the gold and forming a cylinder, as Dr. Dorrance described this afternoon, I take a piece of platinum foil and slip it over the end. Then I take an ordinary bicuspid tooth, or any other, as the case may be, put it on, take a burnisher and burnish it on. I then lay it on a piece of charcoal and heat it. I then use my gold and solder the tooth. It is a very quick and effective way of making a ferule. I have also found it unnecessary to use a blow-pipe in making ferules. I take them in the pliers and hold them over an ordinary Bunsen lamp. It will solder them. I burnish the ends together, and then over the flame of an ordinary Bunsen lamp the solder can be melted right down.

DR. CLAWSON—I find in a great many cases my solder is very brittle and does not flow readily. I have taken a great deal of pains with it, but in a number of instances I have had considerable difficulty. I would like to ask Dr. Talbot if he has had the same difficulty?

DR. TALBOT—Where the solder is brittle I think it is often due to the brass wire that is used, which is not always of the best quality. The wire that I use is very fine, the finest that I can get in the shops.

DR. DORRANCE—I believe the last formula of Dr. Richmond is, coin gold, nine parts, brass wire, two parts, and copper one part. The addition, however, of the brass wire often results in a brittle alloy, for the reason that the arsenic has not been removed from the zinc which is used in the manufacture of the brass. I use a formula which I like very well, and which was given to me by Dr. Robinson. The alloy is made of pure copper, pure silver and pure zinc. If you do not use pure zinc you have a brittle solder. If you use pure zinc you will have a solder which you can roll out, bend double and straighten again, which I think is owing to the fact that there is no arsenic in it. This alloy is good, not only for gold, but also for silver solder. I use from 15 to 30 per cent. To alloy gold, you can make any degree of alloy you wish.

DR. FIELD—In preparing an alloy of this kind, the gold should be melted first and the baser metals dropped in afterward.

DR. DORRANCE—That is a matter which all metal workers know must be done. The metal which melts at the highest temperature must be melted first.

AN ALLEGORY.

BY DR. J. A. ROBINSON.

One day while drowsing till I almost slept,
Some shapeless visions o'er my senses crept,
And took the forms of things I did not know,
And passed and re-passed o'er my slumbering brow.

These shadowing somethings seemed in forms of men,
And then as walking trees appeared again.
I heard loud talks, and arguments arose ;
The noises sounded as if they came from blows.
From all that I could gather, hear, or see,
This war was bred in aristocracy.
Kindly disputes are very good, we know,—
Disputes are only things to make us grow.
We see it everywhere, as we improve,
Innovations only express our love.

I looked again and saw a little stream
Of water, running down a deep ravine.
It ran so quietly along the shade,
I heard the words the gurgling water said.
She said a great, high mountain, changed her course
Over some craigs, her waters to divorce ;
Bade her behold his mountain, he was tall,
While she was insignificant and small.
It was a mountain quarrel with a river.
Which was, to man, the best and greatest giver,

This little modest brook looked very pale,
The stream scarced moved at all, it was so frail,
But still she begged the mountain to withhold,
And even hinted he was getting bold,
When he was talking of his noble calling,
Perhaps he'd need her to prevent his falling.
When he assumed that he could live without her,
If he would listen, he no more would doubt her.

She told him all his grandeur would decay
If she withheld her waters day by day;
If all her streams should wither up and dry,
His grand old forests would decay and die.
Still he was arrogant and bold, and said
He would not stop if everything was dead.

He said he fed the cattle and the sheep,
And grew the grass while they were fast asleep.
He furnished man with iron, coal and wood,
And grew him venison—most delicious food.
He gave him skins of buffalo and bear,
Silver-gray foxes, wolf, and coon and hare;
From his dark womb came forth the shining gold;
The treasures of his breast were manifold.
He wooed the bears and foxes for his brides;
The brooks ran gaily down his mountain sides;
The everlasting pines adorned his head;
The clouds o'er him their silver mantle spread.
He swept foul air from off the weary plain,
Beat it in swirls, till it was pure again.
He felt the rainbow's kiss, the clouds' embrace;
The stupid mule o'er him his path did trace,
With every mineral used to make a nation,
And raise the world to more exalted station.
He taught mankind by symbols in his trees;
Change and decay he taught in every breeze;

In the green woods he taught the general strife
Of man, as he was struggling for life.
The weak and puny raised its little head,
But flourished best when its compeers were dead.
In fruit trees he saw men of real worth;
The elm, his pride and vanity called forth.
He saw in oaks the merchant, rich and strong,
Like small oaks, some were struggling along.
The heads of some looked fierce; their boughs were bent,
They seemed like men who wanted ten per cent.
He saw in poplars, dandies, straight and proud.
In small trees he saw children—quite a crowd.
Where'er the whirlwind or the axe was rife,
He saw the young cut down in prime of life.
He saw a tree all leafless in a field,
Which taught that man was forced by death, to yield.
Although he looked to man, so very tall,
He was made up of particles, very small.
The valleys, where they grew their corn and hay,
Were made so rich, by what he cast away.

The river said he need not feel so grand,
As he acknowledged he was made of sand!
He could not even move beside the shore,
Where he could hear the grand old ocean's roar,
While she could travel over earth and main,
Distil in dew, or gently fall in rain.

In her young life when she was very small
She gaily danced over a waterfall,
And curling 'round into a little nook
She gently grew into a running brook.
She watered all the flowers along the way,
And sailed the boats, for little boys to play.
The fishes jumped, and scud, and whirled about,
And anglers silent crept to fish for trout.
Her flowers grew so bright, her grass so green,

No place so beautiful, was ever seen.
The oaks and willows clustered near the spot,
And lovers vowed their dear forget-me-not.
She ran so gently in this quiet shade,
The little child was not at all afraid.
'Mid moss and grass she gave a sudden whirl,
And was a mirror for an Indian girl!
She watered all the cattle by the way;
Reflected back the sun, brighter than day,
And then she grew so large that she could float
A light canoe or little tiny boat.
Another river came to help her then,
And then she run the factories for the men.
Although her waters did the toiler bless,
She watered all the flowers none the less.
Then she became so deep, and broad, and strong,
She carried sail and steam boats all along.
The rafts, and boats, and sloops, and sailors, seem
As though it was a midnight fairy's dream.
Soon she became a river, fierce and wide,
And nearer to the ocean, and the tide.
Large ships she now upon her bosom carries
As she her waters to the ocean marries.

I looked again; (perhaps it is digression,)
I saw some members of a skilled profession
Trying to cut the handsome thing in two.
While others said they thought it would not do.
Some *aged* members thought they could not see
How we could do so, and have unity.

I saw a marble statue, truly formed,
Resembling mind and body, well adorned
With rounded limbs, and trunk without a spot,
And intellect all pure, and free from blot.
I then beheld the pure and polished stone
Cut, mar'd and hacked, and all its beauty gone.

The marble rough, and soiled, and torn away;
The form and features crumbling to decay.
I thought I saw a glimmer of the way
We should appear, with one half thrown away!

The picture was reversed. I saw a form
Capacitated to be grown upon.
I saw our great professional ideal
Growing, and clothed upon, till it was real.
I saw some sculptors—a strong, valiant band—
With chisel and a mallet in their hand,
Carving from out the world their great ideal,
And fostering our profession, till 'twas real.

The sculptors names' were Tucker, Taft, and Watt,
And hundreds more that I have most forgot,
Tugging away to make it fit to be
A help and blessing to humanity.
Thought after thought, these sculptors, grand and bold,
Gave to the world, ideals to behold!
Higher and higher still they made them rise;
The world, astonished at their sacrifice,
Saw the bright genial warmth of glowing mind,
Leaving old prejudices far behind,
And, like the carvers in the stone, displace
Unwholesome roots, to beautify the face
With artificial dentures, that defy
Detection by the most experienced eye,
As well as saving natural teeth and crowns,
To re-create. where ugliness abounds.
In all departments, everything was fair
And beautiful, for unity was there.
I read the story of the king of old,
What Solomon had said, when he was told
Two women each, had claimed the self-same child,
And how the *real* mother was so wild;

When Solomon had said unto the two,
"Let one half be for her, and half for you."
But when the sword was brought, for deed so foul,
The *real* mother, in her inmost soul
Gave up her child, still, knowing it was wrong,
Saved her child whole—and thus I end my song.

HISTORY OF DENTISTRY IN MICHIGAN.

BY DRS. METCALF AND BENEDICT, COMMITTEE.

GENTLEMEN:—

We are gathered here to-night upon the most auspicious occasion in the history of dentistry in this State. It is not only an event of the deepest interest to our Association, but it marks an important epoch in its history. After a little more than a quarter of a century of associated effort, it is very proper that we should pause for a while, turn back the pages of our record and review the past.

As the careful business man closes his door from the inside and pulls down the shutters that he may inventory his stock, balance his ledger and make plans for the future; or, as in the secret chambers of our hearts each one reviews his own past and brings it all before the tribunal of his conscience, and looks to the future with a resolution for better deeds, so may we pause here, and for a while indulging in reprospect, carefully determine whether our meetings have redounded to our benefit; or, indulging in prospect, may wisely determine *what there is left for us to do* for the elevation of our profession, and for the benefit of mankind.

Your Committee having traced the history of dentistry in this State, over a period of more than half a century of the past, it will be impossible in the time at our disposal this evening, to present to you anything like a narration of events concerning our profession, covering all these years. We shall, therefore, only attempt a respectful mention of a few of the more prominent pioneers of the profession in our State, and then give you such an epitome of the organization and proceedings of this Association, as the hour will permit.

The first practitioner of dentistry in this State, of whom we have any knowledge, was Dr. Douglass Houghton, who commenced practice in the city of Detroit, in 1831. All who are familiar with the early history of Michigan, are familiar with the life of this scholarly and accomplished man; but that our records may have a place inscribed to his memory, I append the following very brief account of his life, which we have gathered from several different sources:

Dr. Douglass Houghton, was born in Troy, N. Y., September 21, 1809, and educated at the Rensslaer Institute, in his native place, and from which he graduated in 1827. The following year he was appointed professor of chemistry and natural history, in the Institute, and while occupying this position he came to Detroit, by request of the citizens, to deliver a course of lectures on scientific subjects. In 1831, he commenced the practice of dentistry in Detroit, and while thus engaged, received a license to practice medicine, from which time, except one or two intervals, he practiced dentistry and medicine, until 1837, when he was appointed Geologist for the State. In 1832, Dr. Houghton was appointed surgeon and botanist to the expedition sent out under Schoolcraft to determine the course of the Mississippi river, which resulted in the discovery of its origin in Itasca lake, on July 13, of that year. From the time of his appointment as Geologist of the State until the time of his death he continued faithfully to discharge the laborious and important duties intrusted to him, developing the resources of the State, and especially in attracting attention to its mineral wealth. In 1842, he was elected mayor of Detroit, and was one of the professors of the University from the time of its organization. He was drowned in lake Superior, near the mouth of Eagle river, during a violent storm, October 13, 1845.

It is worthy of remark in this connection, that when Gen.

Lewis Cass made his first visit to Detroit, after his return to this country from his mission to the court of Louis Phillippe, Dr. Houghton delivered the address of welcome, and when in the fall of 1845, the melancholy news was received of the death of Dr. Houghton, that eminent devotee of science, the meeting which was called to express the sense of public bereavement, was addressed by Gen. Cass, as the principal speaker.

In relation to his ability as a dentist, we have no positive knowledge; but judging from his capabilities in whatever he undertook, we have a right to infer that he was fully equal to those of his time.

The next dentist who came to Michigan, of whom we have any information, was Dr. Michael L. Cardell, who came from Philadelphia, and settled in Detroit in the year 1834, and continued in practice until his decease, which occurred in 1850 or '51. The doctor was a man of fine presence, of remarkable social qualities and an excellent dentist; but of his history prior to his settlement in Detroit, we have been unable to gather any facts.

The next in order was Dr. J. L. Ware, who opened an office in Detroit, in 1836. Dr. Ware commenced his career in Cleveland, where he was engaged in the practice of either dentistry or medicine some ten or twelve years prior to his coming to Michigan. In 1837, Dr. Ware induced Dr. J. H. Farnsworth, a student of his, during the last two years of his practice in Cleveland, to come to Detroit and enter into partnership with him; a partnership which continued for three years. In 1845, Dr. Ware sold out to Dr. F. E. Bailey, and moved to N. Y. City, where he continued in practice until his death.

The Detroit city directory of 1845 contains Dr. Bailey's card, which we insert here as something of a curiosity. "Dr. Bailey, from his former experience and uniform success, while soliciting a share of public patronage, has confidence in saying his operations shall be performed in the latest and most approved manner and always with the least possible inconvenience to his patients, and by the use of Dr. Ware's Nerve Destroyer, he is enabled to remove all sensibility in those teeth otherwise too sensitive for filling, and to destroy the nerve when exposed, without pain or injury to the teeth, this in effect rendering his operations *painless*. Office 75 Woodward Ave."

Dr. J. H. Farnsworth, Sr., as has been previously stated, came from Cleveland to Detroit, and entered into partnership with Dr. Ware, in April, 1837. After practicing together for three years, the partnership was dissolved, and Dr. Farnsworth opened an office for himself, and has continued in active practice until the present time; a continuous practice in the city of Detroit, of *forty-five years!*—during which time he has maintained a reputation of being one of the best operators in the profession.

It would no doubt be interesting to many of you to continue along down the list of early practitioners until we come to the organization of this association in 1855, but the time will permit only mention of the names of a few that followed, and the dates.

Soon after Dr. Ware left Detroit, Dr. C. F. Knowlton, came on from Ohio, and formed a partnership with Dr. Bailey. In 1847, Dr. Bailey sold his interest in the partnership to Dr. W. P. Meacham, of Ohio,—Dr. Bailey returning to that State. Dr. Meacham was a graduate of Gambia Medical College, and a dental student of Dr. John A. Harris, brother of Chapin A. Harris, of Baltimore, author of "Principles and Practice of Dental Surgery." Dr. Meacham never learned to make artificial dentures, but devoted himself entirely to operative dentistry. If living now, he would undoubtedly be an earnest and valuable advocate for "dental divorce," or the separation of professional from mechanical dentistry. It is said of him that he was one of the best operators of his day. Dr. Benedict informs me that in one of his teeth there is now a good filling put there by Dr. Meacham in 1846.

Probably the first dentist in the interior of the State, was Dr. Joseph Mansfield, who located at Niles, in 1837 or '38. Beyond this fact we have been unable to procure any reliable information respecting the early years of his practice.

In the fall of 1839, Dr. L. S. Hotchkiss, now a resident of West Haven, Conn., came from Philadelphia to Michigan, and stopping first at Ann Arbor, commenced an itinerancy that lasted something over a year.

In his letter to the committee, the doctor says: "I commenced the study of dentistry with Dr. Wildman, of Philadelphia, in 1837. In the fall of 1839 I became acquainted with a man from Battle Creek, Michigan, who was in the city purchasing goods. He informed me there had never been a dentist in Michigan west of Detroit, and I thought I could do well in the interior towns. Being full of vitality and venture, I concluded to make the trial. Went by stage and canal to Buffalo, and lake to Detroit, where I stopped one day. Got a ride with a farmer from Detroit to Ypsilanti, in a lumber wagon.

Arriving at Ann Arbor, concluded to make an attack on the defenceless people of that town, so put out my sign and bills. Stopped at the hotel—the only one in town—kept by a man by the name of Pettie. Remained there two or three weeks and did very well. Then went to Marshall, then to Battle Creek, thence to Kalamazoo, visiting each one of these places twice during the winter.

I am quite positive that no one had ever practiced dentistry west of Detroit; certainly not west of Ann Arbor, in Michigan, before me. I heard of one man who had set pivot teeth, made of sea-horse ivory, at Ann Arbor, but he did not fill teeth. I think his name was Farnham, or something like that. He became mixed up in a railroad war, and was sent to State prison. Of course he couldn't have been much of a dentist, or he would have gotten out of a little scrape like that.

The next spring I went to Grand Rapids by stage, which was a lumber box wagon, and I the only passenger. There was no road, only a trail through the woods. We were two days on the trip, stopping over night at a log house.

Remained at Grand Rapids two or three weeks, then went down the river on a steamboat to Grand Haven. From there, crossed the lake to Chicago, on a schooner loaded with lumber. Chicago at that time was not much larger than Kalamazoo. I have always been very glad that I didn't purchase half the town, as it would have burdened me with care, and probably ruined a good dentist.

I left Chicago by stage—a lumber box wagon—another man and myself the only passengers, passed through Michigan City, Laporte, Adrian and Toledo, thence by lake to Cleveland, stage to Pittsburgh, and then by canal most of the way to Philadelphia."

It would be a pleasing task to mention in detail all the pioneer dentists of the interior of the State, and relate the many curious incidents in connection therewith, but in a paper of this length, that will be impossible, and leave room for a review of the proceedings of our association. We shall, therefore, step over a period of fifteen years, without further comment, and come at once to the first convention of Michigan dentists.

In those early days of which we have been speaking, there existed very little, if any, social or professional bond between the members of the profession. They were not only unsocial and uncongenial spirits in each other's presence, but were as shy of each other as a saint is naturally shy of a sinner. Knowledge of methods and processes of the art were treasured as secrets, and every little improvement was usually locked in the discoverer's breast as something sacred to his personal benefit. As an illustration of this tendency to withhold from others any new method or improvement, we relate a little circumstance that occurred as late as 1851. A dentist from one of the southern states—Georgia, we believe—while on a visit to relatives in a little village of Oneida county, N. Y., filled some teeth for them, which happened to fall under the eye of Dr. White, a dentist in the city of Utica. The fillings were so superior to any that had been seen in that vicinity before, that Dr. White resolved to learn the method. Without much loss of time he invested in livery and proceeded to the village where the operator was visiting, and sought his acquaintance, but neither polite attentions, convincing arguments, nor the offer of a generous pecuniary consideration were sufficient to uncover the secret.

An exposed nerve—that tiny filament with which we have all wrestled, and which has defied at times the wisdom of every dentist who has tried to make friends with it,—divulged the great secret. Soon after the southern dentist left for his home, one of his patients, who had a filling that pressed too closely upon the rights of the nerve, walked into Dr. White's office one day with a face that looked like an exaggerated Jack-o-lantern. The extraction of the tooth produced at least a two-fold benefit; it relieved one man of his pain, and another of his secret. It was a *cylinder filling*, and probably the first one that had ever been seen, and for aught I know, ever heard of, in Utica. (It is no part of our duty in the preparation of this paper, to discuss modes or materials, but if we were to-night asked this question: Which is the best form of gold for filling cavities in teeth, we should answer thus: After an observation and experience of thirty-five years, we have found nothing that answers a better purpose, where it can be used to advantage, than soft foil cylinders, properly manipulated.)

While a narrow exclusiveness among dentists, was the general rule, there were a few noble exceptions. Prominent among those who did not believe in that character of secrets which retarded the growth and development of a noble profession, and which withholds from mankind any means calculated to relieve human suffering, were Drs. Whiting and Benedict.

These gentlemen came to Detroit the same year—1847—but from different States.

Dr. L. C. Whiting commenced the study of his profession at Palmyra, N. Y., in 1840, and the same year cast his first vote, which was for Henry Clay, and lost his last dollar on election.

In 1843, he started out to carve his fortune, commencing at Dansville; but after a six weeks trial, became convinced there were some things he did not know, even in dentistry. He returned to his preceptor at Palmyra—who was a brother—and with commendable humility, started in for more light in the profession. In 1845, he opened an office at Port Hope, Ca., remaining two years, and from thence came to Detroit, in 1847, going into the office of his brother, Orson Whiting, who had preceeded him.

Dr. Hiram Benedict, commenced his dental studies in 1845, at Mount Vernon, Ohio, in the office of Dr. W. P. Meachem. He came to Detroit in 1847, and entered the office with Dr. C. F. Knowlton, with whom he remained most of the time, until he entered into a partnership with Dr. Whiting, in 1852.

The office of Drs. Whiting and Benedict, soon became the head quarters for dentists from all parts of the State, when in Detroit. Oftentimes these gentlemen suggested to these visitors, the great amount of good that might be accomplished by a meeting of all the dentists in the State, for the purpose of comparing modes of practice, and the consideration of many matters of interest to the profession. In the fall of 1855, having received sufficient encouragement in the way of promises to attend, they issued the call for a meeting to be held at their office on the evening of January 8, 1855. Here is the tableau of those who responded to the call:

Drs. L. C. Whiting, Hiram Benedict, R. V. Ashley, and C. F. Knowlton, of Detroit; F. M. Foster, Jackson; G. W. Stone, Albion; C. B. Porter, Ann Arbor; T. D. Ingersoll, Monroe; J. J. Jeffries, Lansing; Wm. Cahoon, Pontiac; I. Douglass, R. S Bancroft, Romeo; A. T. Metcalf, Kalamazoo.

A temporary organization was effected by the election of Dr. R V. Ashley, Chairman, and Dr. G. W. Stone, Secretary. After a brief discussion in relation to the expediency of forming a permanent organization at that time, the question was put to vote and decided in the affirmative. On motion, a committee consisting of Drs. Porter, Whiting, Metcalf,

Cahoon and Stone, was elected to prepare a constitution and by-laws for a State Dental Association, and report at 10 o'clock the next morning.

At the meeting, Thursday morning, Dr. Ashley was not present, and Dr. Knowlton was called to the Chair. Indeed, it was soon apparant that Dr. Ashley had turned "the cold shoulder" towards us at the most critical time—just as the convention was about to begin its actual travail in bringing forth a puny child with a big name! We remember distinctly that the report of the committee on constitution and by-laws was severly criticised, and not adopted until after a long discussion and numerous amendments. It was late in the afternoon when by the payment of two dollars each, and signing the constitution and by-laws, that the Michigan State Dental Association was formally organized. The following officers were then elected: President, Dr. C. F. Knowlton; Vice President, Dr. A. T. Metcalf; Recording Secretary, Dr. F. M. Foster; Corresponding Secretary, Dr. L. C. Whiting; Treasurer, Dr. Hiram Benedict. The executive committee and the officers of the association were made a committee to prepare a code of prices for dental operations, a copy to be forwarded to each member of the association, by the 1st of February, proximo, and reported for the action of the next meeting. Drs. Jeffries, Cahoon and Whiting, were appointed to prepare papers on subjects of their own selection.

A vote of thanks was tendered to Drs. Whiting and Benedict for their many courtesies during the meeting, and for the use of their office, and at a late hour on Thursday night the Association adjourned, to convene in the first annual session in the city or Detroit, on Wednesday January 12th, 1857, at 7 o'clock, P. M.

Thus briefly, we give you an account of the organization of this association.

Numerically, the first meeting was not a great success. There were present only thirteen, in all! But they more than fulfilled the purpose for which they assembled. Their actions were characterized by an earnest zeal and devotion to the cause in which they had engaged, that faltered at no discouragement, and which has resulted in accomplishing more than the most sanguine of that little coterie could at that time, have anticipated.

Although more than a quarter of a century has been added to the sum of our years since that little band assembled for the purpose of deliberating for the future good of the profession in our State, nearly all of them still live, and by the mercy of a kind Providence, are here to-night, living witnesses of the growth and prosperity of the Association.

Two have died; Dr. R. V. Ashley, and Dr. J. J. Jeffries.

Dr. Ashley, who was the first temporary chairman of the convention, came to Ypsilanti, this State, from the State of New York, when quite a young man. In 1841 or '42, he entered the office of Dr. Fry, of that place, and soon after completing his studies, purchased the office of his preceptor. He continued in practice at Ypsilanti, until 1851, when he opened an office in Detroit, where he continued in practice until his death, which occurred October 6, 1871, at the age of 62 years. Dr. Ashley was considered an excellent dentist, and secured a remunerative practice.

Dr. Jeffries was a student in the office of Dr. Cahoon. He commenced practice in Lansing, in the fall of 1855, and continued there until 1859, when he gave up the profession. In 1862, he enlisted as a soldier in the 14th Michigan Infantry, and at the time of departure from the State, was captain of his company. He died near Lookout Mountain, in Tennessee, July 19, 1863, of a disease of the bowels. At the time of his death he was a member of Gen. Rosencrantz's staff.

Of the eleven still living, who attended the first meeting, Drs. Whiting, Benedict, Douglass, Bancroft, Porter, Cahoon and Metcalf, are with us to-night.

Drs. Cahoon and Foster gave up the practice of dentistry years ago, for employment more agreeable or remunerative, but they have never ceased to take an active interest in all new developements and improvements, and in the growth and prosperity of the Association.

At the first annual meeting of our Association, held in Detroit, January 7, at 7 o'clock P. M., the President and Vice President were both absent, and Dr. Bancroft was called to the Chair. After the appointment of Drs. Mansfield, Whiting and Porter, a committee to present subjects for discussion, the meeting adjourned until 9 o'clock Thursday morning. The morning came, but no quorum, and another adjournment was had until evening.

The evening session was called to order by Dr. Bancroft, when they proceeded to the election of officers, with the following result: President, Dr. Mansfield; Vice-President, Dr. Foster; Recording Secretary, Dr. Whiting; Corresponding Secretary and Treasurer, Dr. Benedict.

The committee appointed to report subjects for discussion, presented the following list: (1) Cavity plates. (2) Springing of plates. (3) Bending plates. (4) Making solder. (5) Refining gold filings. (6) Alloying gold. (7) Extracting teeth. (8) Treatment of exposed pulps. (9) Destroying nerves. (10) Treatment of alveolar abscess. (11) Dental fees. (12) Making casts. (13) Best material for casts. (14) Taking impressions. *Only* fourteen subjects? The record says: "A promiscuous discussion was then entered into by all the members present, on most of the subjects." This meeting adjourned to meet at Jackson, in July following, "the President and Secretary to give three weeks notice."

At the meeting in Jackson, which commenced July 15—the 1st semi-annual—the time was mostly occupied in the discussion of "fang filling" and "filling with Amalgam, Drs. Porter, Foster and Metcalf were made a committee to report at the next meeting a "code of prices."

The fourth meeting convened in Dr. Porter's office in Ann Arbor, on the evening of January 11, 1858. As there was not a quorum present, meeting adjourned till next day—Tuesday—at 9 o'clock.

At the morning session there were present: Drs. Mansfield, (in the Chair) Foster, Porter, Whiting, Bancroft and Metcalf —six in all. Letters were read from Drs. Taft and Watt, T. D. Ingersoll, L. F. Dreyer, F. W. Stone and Messrs. Jones, White and McCurdy, expressing sympathy and regrets.

The communication from Dr. Ingersoll contained a resignation of his membership in the Association. Dr. Bancroft was appointed a committee to correspond with him and inform him that his resignation is not accepted.

Officers elected: Dr. Mansfield, President; Dr. Porter, Vice President; Dr. Metcalf, Recording Secretary; Dr. Whiting, Corresponding Secretary; and Dr. Benedict, Treasurer.

Four new members were elected: Drs. A. F. Barr, G. W. North, S. A. Gerry and Dr. O. M. Carleton. The committee appointed at the last meeting to make a code of prices, submitted their report, which, after a lengthly discussion on practicability of a general fee bill for the dentists of the State, was finally adopted.

This fee bill as reported and adopted was not made a matter of record, and we have been unable to procure a copy; but a member of the committee has placed in our hands, the lists of minimum prices at that time, of leading dentists in several different States, upon which our fee bill was based. We append a few of them, and you can make your own comparisons with present rates.

DETROIT.

Small cavities with gold............................	$ 1 00
Large " "	$ 1 50 to 3 00
Full sets on gold plate............................	100 00 to 125 00

CLEVELAND.

Small cavities............................	$ 1 50 to 2 00
Large "	2 00 to 10 00
Full sets	100 00 to 150 00

ROCHESTER.

Small cavities		$ 1 00
Large "	$ 1 50 to	3 00
Full sets	100 00	

PORTSMOUTH, N. H.

Small cavities	$ 1 00 to	3 00
Large "	4 00 to	10 00
Full sets	100 00 to	150 00

BUFFALO.

Small cavities		$ 3 00
Large "	$ 4 00 to	10 00
Full sets	100 00	

INDIANAPOLIS.

Small cavities		$ 1 00
Large "	$ 2 00 to	10 00
Full sets	100 00 to	130 00

CHICAGO.

Small cavities		$ 2 00
Large "	$ 3 00 to	8 00
Full sets	120 00 to	150 00

TALLAHASSE, FLA.

Small cavities		$ 2 00
Large "	$ 1 50 to	4 00
Full sets	200 00	

AUGUSTA, GA.

Small cavities		$ 5 00
Large "	$ 6 00 to	15 00
Full sets	250 00	

Notwithstanding the adoption of a general fee bill at the meeting, it did not seem to have the desired effect, for the subject of fees was continually being brought before the Association in some shape, to the exclusion of more valuable discussion, until the meeting of 1865, when the subject appears to have received a death blow in the following very sensible and laconic resolution, which was unanimously adopted: "That fees for services rendered would regulate themselves, and would be in proportion to professional standing."

The fifth meeting was held at the office of Drs. Whiting and Benedict, in the city of Detroit, July 11, 1859, President, Vice President and Secretary, absent. Dr. Bancroft was called to the Chair, and Dr. Harris, Secretary *pro tem*, New members elected: Drs. C. E. Bartlett, Battle Creek; R. V. Ashley, J. H. Farmer, T. A. White, Geo. L. Field, C. Brevort and S. C. Smith; also, Dr. C. S. Chittenden of Hamilton, Ca.; J. T. Toland of Cincinnatti, was made an honorary member.

Dr. Mansfield contributed a valuable paper on "The treatment of exposed nerves," which was read by one of the members, and elicited a very animated discussion. Upon the subject of "filling teeth," several members described their various methods. The record states that "a slate and pencil were procured, and the discussion ran into a conversational and illustrative character, and though highly interesting and instructive, is impossible to report." Dr. Chittenden objects to using "annealed pellets," as they make a hard mass, and liable to get loose in the cavity while packing.

On the subject of "Hemorrhage after extraction," each member appeared with a different remedy; we append a few of them: "Tannin and ether on a pledget of cotton"; "Tinct. Myrrh and Camphor on a pledget of cotton, and held in place by a cork and bandage"; "Perchloride of Iron on a pledget of cotton"; "Vinegar and Alum with compress" and "a soft dry sponge packed in cavity."

A great amount of time was taken up in the discussion of "fang filling," which would be both interesting and instructive to us now. We think Dr. Whiting hit the nail on the head in the following words:—"I believe there is a limit to the preservation of diseased fangs, depending somewhat upon the extent of disorganization, and much upon the constitution and habits of the patient. When the periosteum is destroyed, and all the attachments broken up, there is but little hope for success."

"Taking impressions" was the subject of considerable discussion. For the information of our younger members, we will state that very few at that time used plaster for this purpose.

The meeting of 1850, although the fourth annual, was the sixth meeting of the Association. It convened in Detroit, January 10, the President, Dr. Porter, in the Chair. The number of active members was 31.

The Association having now safely passed the trials and vicissitudes incident to infancy, and in a healthy and prosperous condition, may be said to have fairly started upon the road toward a development of its "eye teeth."

From this time on, it will be impossible to refer to details of the several meetings. We can only recur to those matters which are interesting as evidences of advancement, or subjects of more than ordinary importance.

The first mention of "Vulcanite," is found in the records of 1861, Dr. Porter being appointed to prepare a paper on this subject and present it to the next meeting. In 1862, the value of this material was warmly discussed, many claiming it to be vastly superior to a majority of bases. The price for which sets of teeth on rubber were being made, received a good share of discussion. The record states this:—"there is a general feeling that the prices must be kept up, or the profession go down."

Nothing more on the rubber question is found in the records until 1867, when the "demands of the Hard Rubber Co." were discussed at considerable length," and the following resolution adopted:—"That the members of this Association hereby declare that they will not compromise existing difficulties with the American Dental Vulcanite Co." From this time or very soon after, the latter company commenced their pursuit of the members of our profession, hunting them down and hounding them with an unrelenting wickedness. Their insatiable maw for lucre insisted upon having the last dollar of their arbitrary claim, and even craved the "pound of flesh." Knowing the injustice of the patent,—that it was obtained by fraud and sustained by collusion in the courts, associations were organized to resist, by all lawful measures, the unhallowed demands of the Rubber Co. At this point we would gladly close our eyes to all that follows in connection with this subject, but it has been made an important part of our proceedings, and forms a significant epoch in the history of dentistry in this State, and of the whole United States.

In 1872, or early in 1873, the Dentists of the city of Jackson formed an association of this kind, and employed an "attorney," "so called," to defend them.

A State association was soon formed, and the former association merged into it by some means which have never yet been fully and satisfactorily explained; the new association seemed to inherit, as some sort of legacy I suppose, the aforesaid attorney, "so called." Though an officer of the new association (called the "Dental Protective Union,") I must confess it has always been a mystery to me, exactly how, and when, and where, and by what means the aforesaid "so called" was ever legally retained as its attorney. True, we have acknowledged him as such, because he seemed to come to us—seemed to be ours by right of succession or entailment. We counseled with him, and paid him large sums of money, which was contributed by members of the profession, at home and abroad, and for which he gave us "heap big talk," with a sort of organ swell accompaniment, and performed a few cunning legal gymnastics and slight-of-hand performances.

At the meeting of this Association held at Ann Arbor, October 14, 1873, a committee was appointed to confer with the President and Secretary of the said Protective Union, (who were present) in relation to the merits, condition and claims of that association. After a consultation, the committee made a very favorable report, and recommended as follows:—"that the members of this Association should join the "Protective Union," as by so doing they need have no fear of imposition from the Goodyear D. V. Co." A large number of dentists contributed money to assist the Protective Union, and now the aforesaid "so called" is demanding tribute from these persons, as the price of peace. Josiah Bacon is dead, the rubber patent has expired, and the Protective Union is defunct; but the aforesaid "so called" still exists to remind us of those *funny* times.

Indeed, the aforesaid "so called" seems to have inherited the sweet spirit of Josiah, and we seem to have inherited him. He invites us now to "come down" for his "so called" legal services. Like the boy in the old man's apple tree, that we used to read about, who came down when he threatened to throw stones, some have already "come down" and settled Perhaps, if they had looked the ground over, they would have discovered there were no stones to throw; only tufts of grass and *mud.* Of course, the "so called" can throw mud. Any one can do that. And it may sometimes soil and stain for awhile; but it seldom does a permanent injury. I cannot advise others, but as for me, *I do not propose to "come down!"*

At our meeting held in Detroit, in 1862, when the use of vulcanized rubber as a base for artificial dentures was becoming quite general, it was conceded that in this new material, dentistry had received a severe blow. Its easy manipulation, as compared with the metallic bases, opened the door for ignorant and unprincipled individuals to ride into the profession with very little preparation, and no knowledge whatever of the principles of dental surgery. It was evident that something ought to be done to protect the people from the wickedness practiced by this new class of charlatans, whose only knowledge of dentistry was to tear out the natural teeth, many of which might have been saved, and put in their place illy constructed sets of artificial ones set in rubber. From that time the subject of " Dental Quackery" has afforded a continual theme for discussion at nearly every meeting, but so far, with no satisfactory results.

At the meeting of 1867, it was decided to petition the Legislature for the enactment of a law to regulate the practice of dentistry in this State.

The draft of a memorial embodying the sense of the meeting was presented and adopted, and a committee consisting of Drs. Watling, Holmes, Rix, Benedict, Stone, Field and Owen, appointed to bring the subject properly before the Legislature; but the effort concluded in a lamentable failure. Similar efforts have been repeated at least half a dozen times since, and with the same result. During all these years that we have been making earnest, yet modest and conscientious endeavors to secure a law calculated for the best interests of our fellow citizens, we have witnessed other States on every side, enacting the same provisions for the protection of their people, for which we have plead; and the consequence is, tha medical and dental shysters have fled from those States, and dropped down upon Michigan, as hungry locusts forsake an arid plain and swoop down upon green pastures. We are furnished with laws for the punishment of men who destroy life by violence, but no protection from ruined health and a slow, lingering death, caused by ignorant and unprincipled pretenders in the practice of medicine.

It is amazing that an intelligent people permit themselves to be the daily prey of professional "tramps" who infest our State. Like the common tramp, they tell a plausible story, but not by any means, for old cloths and cold victuals.

In a voice that would put to shame the tones of a caliope, they proclaim themselves the possessors of miraculous powers to heal the sick, to cure cripples, and to preserve and supply teeth. The too credulous victims of their wiles, who seek their miraculous service, are generally confronted by the rule of part "pay in advance," and an amount of pay too largely in advance of the charges made by educated and skillful practitioners of medicine, who have business enough and business integrity enough to stay at home and stand by their work and the reputation it gives them. The traveling pretender justifies his demands for pay in advance, because, being a stranger, he does not and cannot know the pecuniary responsibility of his customer. Does his victim take the hint, that he too is ignorant of the pretender's responsibility, and refuse the extortionate demands for *pay*, before the work is done? Not often. The pretender often claims pay in advance, because he expects soon to go elsewhere. Does this provoke his victim to think or enquire why it is that such a worker of miracles must travel from place to place, like a peddler of small wares, instead of building up a business like other honest and competent men, by proving himself to *be* honest and competent? Not at all. Is it not manifest that the Legislature owes a duty to the people of this State to protect them from the ignorance and the rapacity of these professional swindlers?

Our law does not fail to send the man who obtains money under false pretenses, as a felon to prison. Our law does not permit the engineer of a steamer to perform the functions of his profession, until by an examination by a competent board, he has demonstrated his knowledge of his profession and his capacity to perform its duties. Our law does not permit a common school teacher to guide the child in education, until an examination by competent authority has demonstrated the teacher's knowledge. Our law does not permit the lawyer to take a retainer or to act as an attorney, until by examination, he has demonstrated his knowledge of law and his fitness to practice at the bar. Is the practice of medicine, or surgery, or dentistry, less in its importance to human life and limb, to human well-being and comfort, than these enumerated interests which are entrusted only to those who prove their knowledge of them? Is it entirely safe to trust the life of wife and child, or the dental interests of a family to the traveling quack, who travels because he cannot stay? Would you trust an old bulls-eye watch to the care of a traveling tinker? Is life and health and sound members of so much less consequence than old brass?

But it is said that doctors differ; that they disagree in practice; that they are divided into "pathies;" that the State cannot undertake to decide which is right and which is wrong. It is said people must be left to make their own choice, but this is not relevant to the issue. All good doctors of all "pathies," and all good dentists, and all good and intelligent people should and can combine to require this—this if nothing more—that doctors of every name, pathy or degree, shall demonstrate that they have due knowledge of anatomy, of physiology, of chemistry, of surgery, of midwifery and of pathology. If they know these, they may safely be left to practice medicine without any examination on practice, materia medica and therapeutics. And so in every specialty of medical practice, those who engage in them should likewise be examined in all things pertaining to their specialty. If this be required, can we doubt that the miracle workers will cease to alleviate our miseries and our pocket, and that the traveling medical cyclopediæ will either cease to travel altogether, or at least, cease to travel our way?

But it is said that the diploma—the diploma is the evidence of all this required knowledge. The diploma, indeed!—in these days when one can be bought for from five to fifty dollars, from a Buchanan—or any other cannon—or son of a gun—or of Tom Skuce, or any other *excuse!* Why! the diploma *per se*, proclaims the genuine physician or dentist about as much as a peddler's pack and cheek proclaim the merchant. The diploma as a guaranty of professional equipment and character is worth in these degenerate days, about as much as a white necktie and a black coat. Our only safety is, in obliging doctors and dentists, like lawyers and teachers, to give reliable guaranty to every community in which they offer their services, that they *know something about their business.*

The time cannot be far off when the people of our State will realize the absurdity of permitting any one who may choose, to set himself up for a doctor or a dentist, and experiment upon the human system.

We have been led into this little digression by the conviction that it is our duty as good citizens, standing as we do, in a position where we are forced to see the great danger of allowing ignorant persons to practice the healing art, to direct our efforts in securing a law to regulate the practice of medicine. When this is accomplished, a dental law will naturally follow.

The first allusion to Nitrous Oxide Gas, in the meetings of the Association, according to the record, was in 1864. Here are a few of the opinions that were expressed:

Dr. Whiting stated that he had seen it used, but did not approve of it. Dr. Hawes had used it considerably, but since he had seen accounts of death from its use, was very cautious; preferred chloroform. Dr. Porter said that the medical faculty at Ann Arbor did not approve of it, and had discarded it entirely. Dr. Benedict did not approve of it, and quoted chemists to prove that its administration might prove injurious by developing latent disease or creating a new one. Dr. Gerry was somewhat familiar with it, but considered it injurious. Dr. Knapp had used it considerably, but had no doubt that serious cases were liable to arise from its use. Dr. Watling said that the best dentists had not approved it, and the Association ought not to endorse any article that might be even more injurious than chloroform. Dr. Robinson said that its use would get the dentists in a bad way, by making tooth cobblers of them, and induce the extraction of teeth that ought to be saved.

In the meeting of 1866, the subject was again brought before the Association, and its use as an anesthetic for dental operations endorsed by a large majority of the members as the safest, quickest and best.

The first clinical operation before the Association, was at this session of 1864, by Drs. Robinson and Benedict. A special meeting was called in October of the same year, exclusively for clinics. This is the first time the use of the mallet in plugging teeth is alluded to in the record. Dr. Stone says of it: "I have heard and read a great deal about the use of the mallet in plugging teeth, but have never seen its use before. Am satisfied that its value cannot be appreciated until an operation has been witnessed."

The meeting of 1865 was mostly occupied in clinical operations by Drs. Watling, Benedict, Cahoon and others using the mallet and Dr. Metcalf's Annealing Lamp.

By Resolution in 1869, clinical exercises are thereafter excluded from the order of business.

An award of a medal, worth at least $25, was offered by the Association, to any member inventing the best automatic mallet.

During the following two years, several were exhibited, two of them by our members, which were referred to Drs. Benedict, Cahoon and Stone.

At the meeting of 1865, Dr. Robinson called attention to the propriety of memorializing the Regents of the University for the establishment of a dental chair, in the medical department of that institution. The suggestion met with a hasty endorsement, and was acted upon at once, and Drs. Robinson, Field, Cahoon, Porter and Benedict, were appointed a commitee to draft and present to the Regents, a petition, in behalf of the Association. In 1866, Dr. Benedict, in behalf of the committee, reported that they had performed the duty assigned them, and in addition to their instructions, had secured the services of Dr. Taft, of Cincinnatti, to present the memorial. In his report, Dr. Benedict says: the Regents referred the matter to the medical committee, who reported adversely to the plan, for the present, and this report was adopted by the

Regents. A brief and quite informal discussion of the prospect, followed the report of the committee, which to the surprise of all, eliminated a very fair view of a dark object, about the size of a colored gentleman, in the University wood pile. Defeated so far, but not discouraged, Drs. Benedict, Stone and Field were appointed a committee to again "memorialize the Regents of the University, for the establishment of a dental chair." In 1867, this committee, made a verbal report, of which we have no record, and were discharged. The subject was brought up a second time during the session, and the same committee reappointed for the purpose of a conference with the Regents, relative to the prospect. The following year the committee reported "no progress," and were discharged from the further consideration of the subject, and a committee consisting of Drs. Field, Benedict, Holmes, Stone and Bancroft appointed to bring the subject before the next Legislature. So far as the records show, the Association took an absolute rest from any further agitation of this subject for a number of years. In 1872, the project was again brought up. The Association having evidently fully recovered from the demoralizing effect of its former disastrous defeats, took fresh courage, and resolved to renew the attack. Drs. Holmes, Jackson, Hauxhurst, Thomas and Robinson were appointed a committee to confer with the Regents.

In 1873, this committee made a verbal report, in which they stated, that the Regents are not only willing, but would be glad to establish a dental department, as soon as the necessary funds are provided. On motion the committee was continued. Dr. Thomas "urged the necessity of each member of the Association constituting himself a special committee to labor with the representative of his district, to secure an appropriation to establish a dental department in the University."

The next year, 1874—Dr. Holmes, Chairman—committee on a dental department in the University, reported that he found the Professors and Regents in favor of the movement, but the funds were not at hand, suggested the propriety of petitioning the Legislature to collect a special tax for the purpose. Said that nothing further could be done, until the next session of the Legislature, when the committee should labor with that body.

The report of the committee opened the door for a long, and animated discussion, of which the following is the substance as near as we can express it in a few words. Dr. Field opposes the movement; says he thinks we have too many dental colleges to support. Should not establish any new ones until we can support those we have now. That college education does not always make a dentist, and knows of cases where college graduates are a disgrace to the profession. Does not wish to be understood that he opposes a thorough dental education. The reason the colleges do not send out better dentists, is because we do not send good enough students. Thought more colleges would lessen the standard. Dr. Watling thinks that a more thorough preparation to practice dentistry can be obtained at the University, with proper teachers, than at any exclusively dental college. Dr. Jackson thinks we ought to have some place where a thorough knowledge of dentistry can be obtained, before we pass a law to prevent quackery. Dr. Post thought a dental department at our University, would be a great benefit, and recommended continual application, until we meet with final success.

Dr. Thomas fully agrees with Dr. Holmes, that if we are a branch of the medical profession, we ought to be sustained in our effort to get a good education; advocates raising a fund by dentists, to establish a dental department in the University. The only way to turn out thorough dentists, is by a thorough education. Dr. Jackson believed in a full knowledge of medicine, in order to practice dentistry successfully. Dr. Holmes says, dentistry is not a trade, but must be looked up to, as a scientific calling, and hoped we would all take an interest in dental education. Watling says, the strife between colleges is too great to make good practical dentists. Jackson thinks we ought at least to have sufficient knowledge to treat all abnormal conditions of the mouth successfully. Douglass thinks we ought to have a better knowledge of medicine. Dr. Hauxhurst believes we should exert ourselves to gain a higher place in the sciences. Dr. Douglas thinks our surest way to gain a better knowledge of dental education, is to establish a dental department in the University.

When the Legislature of 1875 convened, Dr. Holmes, Chairman of the committee, had a bill prepared, backed by a strong petition of prominent citizens of Grand Rapids, which he placed in the hands of the Hon. E. L. Briggs, representative of the third district of Kent county. It was the last of a series of bills introduced by that gentleman, and he was induced to present it, only upon the assurance, that after it was once before the Legislature, he would be relieved of further care and responsibility regarding it. We append a copy of the bill, as passed.

STATE OF MICHIGAN.

No. 518.

HOUSE OF REPRESENTATIVES.

[INTRODUCED BY MR. BRIGGS.]

A BILL

To provide for an appropriation to enable the board of regents to establish and maintain a dental school in connection with the medical department of the State university.

SECTION 1. *The People of the State of Michigan enact*, That there shall be, and is hereby appropriated out of any funds in the treasury of the State of Michigan, not otherwise appropriated, the sum of three thousand dollars for each of the years 1875 and 1876, for the purpose of enabling the board of regents to establish and maintain a dental school in connection with the medical department of the State university. The above mentioned sum shall be drawn from the treasury, on the presentation of the proper voucher of the treasurer of said board to the auditor general, and on his warrant to the State treasurer.

Passed, April 27, 1876. Yeas, 64. Nays, 19.

This bill, during its incubation, passed through the usual stages of such measures, with various perturbations and spasmodic indications of both failure and success. While it had the united prayers of all the leading dentists in our State, for its support and success, the only ones to be seen in the lobby of the Legislature, at the critical time of birth, were Drs. Finch, of Adrian, and Cole, of Lansing. By their presence at this time, they rendered efficient and valuable service. By the time of our meeting, in October 1875, the arrangements for establishing a dental college, in connection with the medical department of the University, had been completed. That there was joy among the members of this Association on account of the passage of the dental bill, thus terminating the labors and anxieties of years in a triumphant victory, a brief glance at the record of the meeting will abundantly show.

By Dr. E. S. Holmes; Whereas, the "Michigan Dental Association" has labored long and persistently to secure the establishment of a dental department to the University of Michigan; and whereas, the people of the State of Michigan, through their legislative representatives, have enabled the board of Regents to establish such department;—therefore, this Association feeling an ardent desire for the welfare of the school, and a warm interest in its success, prosperity and usefulness, and wishing to express our appreciation of favors shown to the said dental department, do resolve that the thanks of this Association be tendered to Messrs. S. S. White, Philadelphia, Pa.; Buffalo Dental Manufacturing Co., Buffalo, N. Y.; Prittie & Buffum, Detroit, Mich.; Johnson Brothers, New York City; J. R. B. Ransom, Toledo, Ohio; G. W. Archer, Rochester, N. Y.; S. R. Bingham, Chicago, Ill.; Messrs. Lane & Payne, Rochester, N. Y.; Messrs. A. M. Leslie & Co.,

St. Louis, Mo.; Tieman & Co., N. Y.; R. S. Bronson & Son, Buffalo, N. Y.; L. S. Lerch, Ann Arbor, Mich.; Blake & Co., Philadelphia, Pa.; Spencer, Crocker & Co., Cincinnati, Ohio; Codman & Shurtleff, Boston, Mass.; Wm. Johnson, Detroit, Mich., for valuable donations of chairs, tools, appliances and instruments to the University of Michigan, for the use of the department of dentistry. Adopted.

By Dr. Thomas.

Resolved, That a consulting and visiting committee of three, be elected by the "Michigan Dental Association," to confer with the teachers of the dental department of the University, as often, and upon such matters of interest, as may at any time come before them, and such committee to be elected by ballot, the chairman of said committee to be elected for three years, the others, one for two years, and one, for one year, and one member to be elected yearly thereafter. Committee elected: Drs. Metcalf, Thomas and Finch.

By Dr. Parker.

That the Secretary be instructed to prepare and distribute a circular among the profession, soliciting contributions of interesting specimens for the purpose of establishing a museum in connection with the dental department of the University.

By Dr. Spellman.

That an appropriation of one hundred dollars be made from the treasury of this Association to the "University of Michigan," for the use of the dental department.

At the special session called December 13, 1878, for the purpose of taking some action to secure an increased appropriation for a proper maintenance of the dental college, Dr. Thomas makes the following statement:

Students have increased at the rate of an average annual gain of more than 40 per cent., which may fairly be regarded as evidence of permanent growth, and of high appreciation by the profession, in the State and country. Especially encouraging, in view of the fact that the term of study each year is longer then that of any other school in the country, with perhaps, possibly, one exception; while the standard of attainment for entrance into both junior and senior classes, is far higher than that of any other dental college in the land.

What follows in relation to the dental college, is furnished by the kindness of Dr. Taft:

The Regents, though looking upon the project with marked approbation, felt that the financial condition of the University was such at that time, that it would be impossible for them to establish such a department And it seemed too impracticable to attempt it without a special appropriation from the Legislature. And thus the enterprise was stayed for the time being, though not at any time was it abandoned, but it may properly be considered as having been in a state of incubation. The matter thus rested until the winter of 1874—5, when the Legislature in answer to a petition from a large number of people, made an appropriation of $6,000, for establishing a dental college, and carrying on its work for the succeeding two years. The leading members of the profession in Michigan, were much interested, and put forth energetic efforts for the organization of the college. After the appropriation was made, the Regents took prompt action, and proceeded to the establishment and organization of the college.

The minutes of the proceedings of the board of Regents of May 11, 1875, has the following:

On motion of Regent Grant, Dr. E. S. Holmes was invited to address the board, relative to the organization of a dental college in connection with the medical department of the University. Dr. Thomas, Dr. Watling, and Dr. Jackson addressed the board in relation to the same subject.

At the same meeting, the following was unanimously passed;

Resolved, That the college of "dental surgery" be placed under the charge of the committee in the medical department.

On the next day, Wednesday, May 12, the following resolution submitted by Regent Rynd, relative to the organization of a "college of dental surgery," was adopted:

Resolved, That a "college of dental surgery be established, which shall in addition to the facilities now afforded by the medical department, and chemical laboratory, be constituted by the founding of two professorships.

Resolved, That the dental profession of the State be requested to co-operate with the Regents, by suggesting at the June meeting, such names, as they may deem suitable, and also by securing the necessary outfit."

The following was also printed by Dr. Rynd:

Resolved, That the committee on buildings, and the Secretary, be and are hereby instructed to make the necessary arrangements for the furnishing of a lecture room, for the use of the dental college. These resolutions were passed by the unanimous vote of the board.

At the next meeting of the Regents, held June 29, 1875, the following preamble and resolutions of the "Michigan Dental Association" were presented by Regent Rynd, and on his motion were accepted and ordered to be printed in the minutes.

At a special meeting of the "Michigan Dental Association," held in Detroit, May 25, 1875, the following resolutions were adopted:

WHEREAS, The Legislature of the State of Michigan has enacted a law appropriating the sum of $3,000 per year, for the years 1875—6, for the purpose of establishing a dental department in the University at Ann Arbor; be it

Resolved, That the members of the Michigan State Dental Association, fully endorse and approve of the action of the board of Regents of said University at their late meeting, looking toward the establishment of such dental department.

Resolved, further, That we as members of the dental profession, and as individuals, will do all in our power to aid in the establishment and maintenance of such department.

Resolved, That the board of Regents be requested to appoint two professors, [to be suggested by this Asssciation,] one, of dental medicine and surgery, the other, of operative and clinical dentistry.

It was moved and carried, that the Regents be requested by this Association, to invite Professor J. Taft, of Cincinnatti, to accept the professorship in the University of "dental medicine and surgery."

Resolved, That a copy of these resolutions be sent to the Secretary of the Hon. Board of Regents.

At the meeting of the Regents in the afternoon of the same day, Professor C. L. Ford, of the medical department, being present, was requested by the board to make a statement relative to the organization of some of the best dental schools with which he is at present acquainted. At the close of this statement he made the following recommendations:

1st. That there be required three years study in the office of a good dentist, in connection with attendance upon lectures in the University, equal at least to one full course of medical lectures.

2nd. That thorough provision be made for instruction in surgical and mechanical dentistry.

Regent Rynd offered the following:

Resolved, That J. Taft, D. D. S., of Cincinnatti, be and is hereby appointed professor of the Principles and Practice of dental medicine and surgery in the college of dental surgery in the University of Michigan. Salary to be fixed at the next meeting of the board.

Resolved, That the President of the University of Michigan be and is hereby instructed to invite Dr. J. Taft to meet the medical faculty and such other persons as may be officially interested in the establishment of the college of dental surgery.

These resolutions were passed by the unanimous vote of the Board.

The President of the University, in his report to the board of Regents, for the year ending June 30, 1875, says: "A committee charged with power to act, have appointed John A. Watling, D. D. S., Professor of clinical and mechanical dentistry. Further in the report occurs the following statement:

The members of the dental profession in the State, have for some time been desiroūs of securing the establishment of a dental school here. The Regents and their medical faculty here repeatedly expressed to them an earnest wish to co operate with them in attaining their end. The grant of the Legislature enables us to set a school in operation.

There seems good reason to expect for it a successful future. Hardly any similar school in the country furnishes so thorough and extended instruction in those branches of medical science, which are a part of dentists' education, and only one other offers the general advantages of University life to its students. Then there is a large territory near us which is unprovided with such a school. There is none in Illinois, Indiana, Wisconsin, Minnesota or Iowa. If the school prospers, as we may reasonably trust it will, ampler means will be required for its support, and doubtless will be provided.

By these references, it is clearly seen that the dental college had in the beginning, the interest and hearty co-operation of the board of Regents and all the authorities of the University, as well as that of the Profession throughout the State, and this interest and co-operation has been manifested from the beginning to the present hour. In providing accommodation for the college, the building now used by the homeopathic school, which was, previous to that a dwelling, was remodeled and made commodious and convenient for the college, having lecture and clinic rooms, and a laboratory in the basement.

In supplying fixtures, tools and instruments, the Profession of the State and the dealers in dental materials generally, were liberal in contributions; these came unsolicited, and were accepted as an evidence of warm interest in the enterprise A liberal donation of books, were made chiefly by Drs. L. C. Whiting, H. Benedict and B. T. Spellman.

Soon after the organization, an announcement was issued. On October 1, 1875, the 1st term opened with twenty students, quite as large a number as any had ventured to predict. The work of the course was at once commenced, and continued through the six months without interruption or anything to mar its harmony. The special instruction was given by the three teachers already referred to. Of the twenty students present, eleven were from Michigan, three from Ohio, three from Indiana and three from Illinois. In the class of 1876—7, there were thirty-three;—eighteen from Michigan, eight from Ohio, three from Indiana, two from Illinois, one from N. Y. and one from Minnesota. For the next four years there was a steady increase in the number in attendance, as follows: Term of 1877—8, forty-three; 1878—9, sixty-two; 1879—80, eighty-three; 1880—81, eighty-six; and 1881—82, seventy-six. The graduating classes have been as follows:

1876.

D. C. Hauxhurst,	R. H. Tremper,	George J. Carter,
W. H. Jackson,	G. E. Post,	George E. Wright,
A. C. Beecher,	L. L. Davis.	

1877.

M, Holland, M. D.,	P. McGregor,	George S. Shattuck,
William G. Stowell,	V. H. Jackson,	S. B. Hartman,
P. J. Kester,	G. W. Irvin,	J. L. Modgman,
Ulrich Kreit.		

1878.

E. E. Arnold,	William Mitchell,	James B. McGregor,
Thomas S. Ewing,	Alvin Knapp,	William H. Miller,
Sherman F. Finch,	John N. Cowen,	Eben L. Parker,
Fremont E. Lyon,	Mark F. Finley	George H. Wilson,
Benjamin F. Miller,	Charles W. Sanderson.	

1879.

David M. Cattell,	F. Frank Sites,	Edwin J. Lilly,
Frank O. Gilbert,	Corydon L. F. Wall,	Henry B. Orr,

Herbert F. Harvey,	Frank B. Wells,	Samuel B. Short,
James H. Kennicott,	Clark L. Gregory,	Frank H. Waldron,
Howard T. Sackett,	George T. Higgins,	William H. Dorrance.

1880.

William Berry Armendt,
Thomas Wesley Beckwith,
Uriah Dildine Billmeyer,
William Fairman Bradner,
George Hart Brown,
David Ethelbert Callaghan,
John Peter Carmichael,
Suel Erastus Clark,
Williams Donally,
Hiram Edgar Dunn,
Alma W. E. Fuellgraff,
Douglas Potterf,
William John Poyser,
John Nelson Reynolds,
Collins McKnight Roe,
Ira Emmit Sampsell,
Charles Edwin Stroud,
Frank F. Hoyer,
Alfred Wright Hoyt,
Ormand Courtland Jenkins,
Aaron Churchill Johnson,
George Frederick Kimball,
Thomas Chalmers Leiter,
Frank Flavius Little,
Amos Marion Long,
Ossian C. Moon,
Arthur Clayton Nichols,
Evelyn Pierrepont,
Immer C. St. John,
Maurice James Sullivan,
Olin Stacy Voak,
Julius Charles Waldron,
Wilbur Silvius Whisler,
Robert Addison Young,

1881.

George Washington Avery,
Wilbert George Bean,
Henry Franklin Billmeyer,
Albert Victor Bills,
Ephraim David Brower,
Joseph Burger,
Solon Orville Burrington,
Charles Robert Calkins,
George Henry Corey,
Henry C. Corns,
Lewis Craine,
William Milo Hunt,
Augustus Neil Johnson,
Edward Lincoln Kellogg,
Jennie Catherine Kollock,
John James Little,
Charles Maclean,
Guy Hamilton Morgan,
Clarence Doolittle Peck,
Denton E. Peterson,
William Henry Priestman,
Charles Jay Siddall,

Hiram DePuy,
Harry Edgarton,
Alban Vaughan Elliott,
Almos Elias Emminger,
Fred N. Emerick,
Orion Jonathan Fay,
Stephen Humbert Gerow,
Charles A. Sipe,
Arthur Everet Smith,
Joseph William Wassall,
Howard S. West,
B. Clark Williams,
Frank Duane Wilson,
Lawson Deforest Wood.

1882.

Geo. P. Ashton,
Wellington B. Banks,
Frederic J. Barnes,
Fred. T. Bell,
James C. Bush,
Chas. Eckert,
Chas. E. Cleveland,
Margaret Humphreys,
Henry A. Knight,
Joseph D. Little,
Henry M. Loughridge,
Hattie A. Martindah,
Kate L. Moody,
Frank S. Morrison,
Edwin M. Nutting,
Romeyn M. Paine,
John W. Campbell,
Jennie M. Clark,
Edward C. Carditt,
Herbert LuDavis,
Bernard J. DeVries,
Chas. F. Porter,
William U. Biestman,
James W. Lynn,
Joseph L. Rose,
Walter I. Southerton,
Edward Stiles,
Wilbur A. Studley,
Robley Sturgeon,
Henry B. Tileston,
William A. B. Tredway,
James M. Welch.

At the end of the second term, Dr. Jackson resigned his position as Demonstrator of mechanical dentistry, and soon after, Dr Dorrance, of Jackson, was appointed, at a salary of $500. At the end of two years his salary was increased to $800. At the end of the next year, Dr. Watling resigned the Chair of mechanical dentistry, and Dr. Dorrance was appointed Professor of prosthetic and metallurgic dentistry. In June, 1880, Dr. W. D. Billmeyer was appointed assistant in the clinical department. In June, 1881, Dr. C. I. Case, of Jackson, Mich., was appointed assistant in prosthetic dentistry. Dr. C. L.

Ford, Professor of Anatomy, in the medical department of the University, has been a member of the dental college from the organization of the school, to the present, and has performed a very large amount of work each year, for the special benefit of the dental college, which, though highly appreciated, should have been recognized in a more substantial way. The other members of the medical faculty have given special work to the dental classes, whenever their arduous labors in other directions would permit.

The material facilities employed by this department are worthy of mention. Five years ago the college was moved into its present quarters. The western part, or that formerly used as a dwelling, sufficient for the first year, the increase in attendance was such, as to make more room necessary, for the proper prosecution of the work, and in the autumn of 1879, the eastern part of the present building was erected, 64 feet long and 24 feet wide, and two stories high, in which ample accommodation was offered at the time, and it was supposed would be sufficient; but within two years after its erection, its capacity was tested to its utmost. It still reasonably well accommodates the prosthetic department, but more room is now needed for the clinical work. The front room is crowded with thirty chairs, while often, thirty-five are needed. The laboratory and clinic rooms have been fitted with all needed machinery, tools, instruments and appliances for the work to be done in each. The museum contains about $1200 worth of models, preparations and charts for illustration in teaching the various branches. Over $1000 has been invested in models and preparations of the most perfect construction, all of which are of French manufacture. The college has a special library containing over 200 volumes, which contains all the leading works on dental science, with those of recent and earlier dates. Additions are constantly being made as other works are obtainable. The intention is that it shall contain every work published, especially in the English language, on dental science, both direct and collateral. All the dental journals of the

U. S. and England are in the library. The library is open throughout the term for consultation by the students. *The status* of the college may be somewhat estimated by the very generous support given it by the profession of this country, and other countries as well.

The classes have increased from the beginning to the present beyond the most ardent expectations of the founders and friends of the institution, and this too, while the standard of requirements for both entrance and graduation have been from year to year somewhat more stringent, and almost every year has added something to the extent of the curriculum, which has seemed necessary to keep abreast with the progress of the times. Another encouraging feature as to the standing of the college is shown in the fact that its graduates are in demand and sought for by the profession. The close of each term brings many requests for our students, calling them to inviting fields for professional occupation. The fact that the diploma of the college has full recognition in European countries, especially in England, Ireland and Scotland, where a public declaration of such recognition has been made, is an indication not to be mistaken or lightly esteemed.

Almost every subject of interest and importance to the profession during the past ten or twelve years, has received due attention by the association; and as our proceeding for these years are comparatively familiar to you, we will allude to only one or two of them.

At the meeting of 1870, on the subject of "dental education," Dr. Thomas made an excellent speech from which we extract the following:

"I have been fully and thoroughly convinced that operative and mechanical dentistry ought to be separated, as they are two separate and distinct branches of business. A man who devotes a large portion of his time to mechanical dentistry, is wholly unfit for operative dentistry. I believe that just so long as the present system is in vogue, just so long will incompetent dentists be turned out to impose on the public. The profession should take a higher stand and insist upon a thorough education."

At the meeting of 1881—our last session—one of our members exhibited his ignorance and boldness, his impudence and audacity, his simpleness and stupidity by introducing the following resolutions: "That the President of this Association and the Board of visitors to the dental department of the University, are hereby instructed to make all proper efforts to have the Chair of mechanical dentistry abolished."

As might naturally be expected, this endeavor in the direction of a new departure, elicited a very animated discussion here, and in due time "stirred up the animals" all over the country.

Among those who participated in our discussions, Dr. Thomas came to the front with a well guarded speech. In fact, it was so diplomatic, that some doubt seemed to exist as to his position, which brought out Dr. Field with the following pertinent inquiry: "I would like to ask the gentlemen on the floor just now, which side of the fence he is on?" Dr. Thomas then defined his position as being in sympathy with the sentiment of the resolution, but did not believe the time had come yet, when we can dispense with teaching mechanical dentistry in the dental college. During the year, some sense and considerable nonsense has been printed in our dental journals in reference to the resolution and stupidity of the member who introduced it.

It is a source of cheer and of pride also to the author of the resolution, that a large number of the acknowledged leading dentists of the country have rallied to his support in letters of congratulation and endorsement, and he is confident the day is not far distant, when the resolution may be taken from the table where it now sleeps, to usher in an era of standing and dignity due to a scientific profession, and those who practice as DOCTORS OF DENTAL SURGERY.

NOTE.

The association express regrets that Drs. Metcalf, Field, Thomas, J. Lathrop, Cowie and Robinson, could not be in attendance only at the evening sessions; as they were obliged to attend Circuit Court. Drs. Metcalf and Robinson as witnesses, the other named as defendants in a suit brought by C. C. Burt, an alleged lawyer, to collect a fee of Fifteen Thousand Dollars, for services rendered a number of years ago. However, the suit was finally thrown out of court, and a judgment which he had previously obtained, set aside on the ground that said Burt had no case against these gentlemen. The litigation was brought to a close in time for those interested to enjoy the festivities of the Quarter Century Banquet, with a decided relief to their minds and pockets.

REDUCED PRICES ON TEETH.

WHITE'S AND JUSTI'S.

	Gum	Plain
For Single Teeth, - -	Gum, 15c. each.	Plain, 10c. each
For $15 00 Cash, - -	" 14 "	" 9½ "
For 25 00 " - -	" 13 "	" 9 "
For 50 00 " - -	" 12½ "	" 8½ "
For 100 00 " - -	" 12 "	" 8 "

NEALL'S, TANTUM'S AND SIBLEY'S.

Single Tooth, Gum or Plain,			$ 08
Per Sets of 14's,		"	1 00
12	"	"	10 00
25	"	"	20 00
31	"	"	25 00
63	"	"	50 00
130	"	"	100 00

5% Discount for Cash on $50 00 lots of goods, except Teeth at quantity prices, and Precious Metals.

10% Discount for Cash on $150 00 lots of goods, except Teeth at quantity prices, and Precious Metals.

Akron Rubber,	Per lb.	$3 00
Sampson "	"	3 00
Doherty's, "	"	2 50
Bowspring "	"	3 00
Black "	"	2 50
Weighted "	"	4 00
English Pink Rubber,	"	7 00

AMALGAMS, all kinds, - - - - $2 00 to $5 00 per oz.

MICHIGAN GOLD AND PLATINA ALLOY, best in the market, Per oz., $3 00

"GOLD FOIL," "CYLINDERS," "PELLETS, &C."

White's, Hood & Reynolds', Williams', Ney's, Pack's, Kearsings, &c. Per ⅛ oz., $4 00. Per ½ oz., $15 00. Per oz., $30 00.

NICKOLDS' ADHESIVE GOLD. Per ⅛ oz., $3 75. Per ½ oz., $14 00. Per oz., $28 00.

NICKOLDS' IMPROVED SOFT GOLD. Per ⅛ oz., $4 00. Per ½ oz., $15 00. Per oz., $29 00.

We allow Students in attendance at Colleges, and for three months after graduating, 10% off for cash.

We have constantly on hand, SECOND HAND ENGINES, CHAIRS, &c., of which we will send prices, etc., on application.

Refilling Gas Cylinders, 100 gallons, - - - - $6 00
" " 500 " - - - - - Per gal., 4½c.

Charges paid one way by us.

METAL TOP TOOTH POWDER BOTTLES.

Plain Round,	Per doz., 75c.
Fancy,	" 80c.

ABSORBENT COTTON.—Extra Fine.

One-half ℔ packages,	60c.
One-quarter ℔ "	35c.
Two oz. "	20c.

FLOSS SILK.—A very Superior Article.

Plain,	Per doz., $1 50	Per spool, 15c.
Waxed,	" 2 25	" 20c.

FRENCH POLISHING STRIPS, very thin, - - - Per box, 50c.

PHENOL SODIQUE, - - - - - - Per bottle, 50c.

FRENCH'S SELECTED DENTAL PLASTER.

Per barrel, full 300 ℔s.,	$5 00
Per one-half barrel,	3 25
Per keg,	2 25
Per ℔. in packages,	3

REDUCTION IN PRICE.

Nickel Plated Forceps,	Per pair, $2 25
Banner Amalgam,	Per oz., 2 00

It is to the interest of **every Dentist in Michigan,** to have a first-class Dental Depot in their own State, and the more you help us the larger stock we can keep, and the better we can fill your wants.

Send your **mail** orders **direct** to us, and we will try and please you.

REDUCED PRICES ON TEETH.

WHITE'S AND JUSTI'S.

	Gum	Plain
For Single Teeth,	Gum, 15c. each.	Plain, 10c. each
For $15 00 Cash,	" 14 "	" 9½ "
For 25 00 "	" 13 "	" 9 "
For 50 00 "	" 12½ "	" 8½ "
For 100 00 "	" 12 "	" 8 "

NEALL'S, TANTUM'S AND SIBLEY'S.

Single Tooth, Gum or Plain,			$ 08
Per Sets of 14's,		"	1 00
12	"	"	10 00
25	"	"	20 00
31	"	"	25 00
63	"	"	50 00
130	"	"	100 00

5% Discount for Cash on $50 00 lots of goods, except Teeth at quantity prices, and Precious Metals.

10% Discount for Cash on $150 00 lots of goods, except Teeth at quantity prices, and Precious Metals.

Akron Rubber,	Per lb. $3 00
Sampson "	" 3 00
Doherty's, "	" 2 50
Bowspring "	" 3 00
Black "	" 2 50
Weighted "	" 4 00
English Pink Rubber,	" 7 00

Amalgams, all kinds, - - - - $2 00 to $5 00 per oz.

Michigan Gold and Platina Alloy, best in the market, Per oz., $3 00

"Gold Foil," "Cylinders," "Pellets, &c."

White's, Hood & Reynolds', Williams', Ney's, Pack's, Kearsings, &c. Per ⅛ oz., $4 00. Per ½ oz., $15 00. Per oz., $30 00.

Nickolds' Adhesive Gold. Per ⅛ oz., $3 75. Per ½ oz., $14 00. Per oz., $28 00.

Nickolds' Improved Soft Gold. Per ⅛ oz., $4 00. Per ½ oz., $15 00. Per oz., $29 00.

We allow Students in attendance at Colleges, and for three months after graduating, 10% off for cash.

We have constantly on hand, SECOND HAND ENGINES, CHAIRS, &c., of which we will send prices, etc., on application.

Refilling Gas Cylinders, 100 gallons, - - -	$6 00
" " 500 " - - - - -	Per gal., 4½c.

Charges paid one way by us.

METAL TOP TOOTH POWDER BOTTLES.

Plain Round, - - - - - -	Per doz., 75c.
Fancy, - - - - - - -	" 80c.

ABSORBENT COTTON.—Extra Fine.

One-half ℔ packages, - - - - - - -	60c.
One-quarter ℔ " - - - - - -	35c.
Two oz. " - - - - - -	20c.

FLOSS SILK.—A very Superior Article.

Plain, - - - -	Per doz., $1 50	Per spool, 15c.
Waxed, - - - -	" 2 25	" 20c.

FRENCH POLISHING STRIPS, very thin, - - -	Per box, 50c.

PHENOL SODIQUE, - - - - - -	Per bottle, 50c.

FRENCH'S SELECTED DENTAL PLASTER.

Per barrel, full 300 lbs., - - - - - - -	$5 00
Per one-half barrel, - - - - - -	3 25
Per keg, - - - - - - -	2 25
Per ℔. in packages, - - - - - -	3

REDUCTION IN PRICE.

Nickel Plated Forceps, - - - - -	Per pair, $2 25
Banner Amalgam, - - - - -	Per oz., 2 00

It is to the interest of **every Dentist in Michigan,** to have a first-class Dental Depot in their own State, and the more you help us the larger stock we can keep, and the better we can fill your wants.

Send your **mail** orders **direct** to us, and we will try and please you.

REDUCTION IN PRICES.

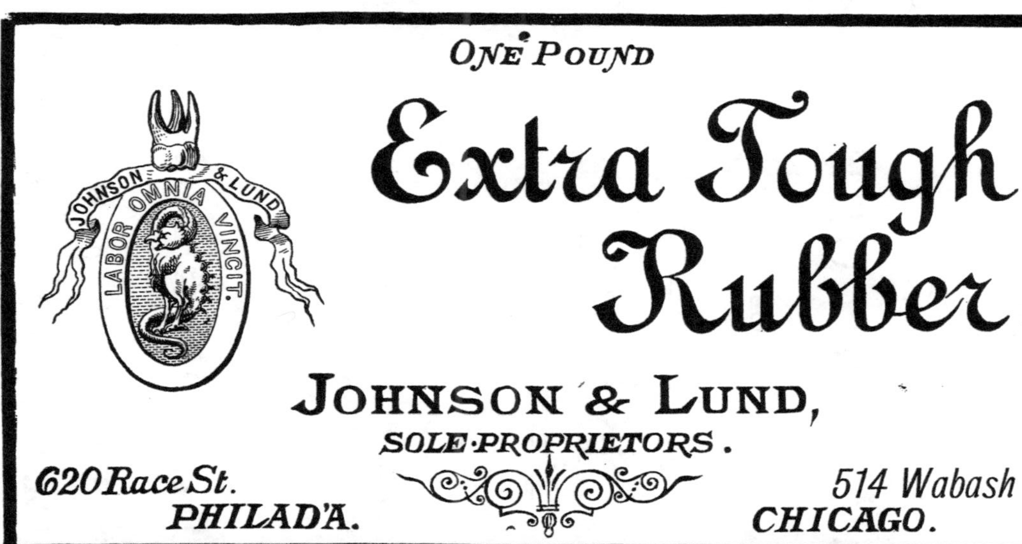

PRICES.

Per Single Pound,
$3.00

Per 5 Ponnd Lots,
$2.70 Lb.

Per 10 Pound Lots,
$2.40 Lb.

Per Sheet, 20c.

Registered in the Patent Office at Washington, Nov. 21st, 1874.

The EXTRA TOUGH RUBBER is offered to the profession with the assurance that its good qualities place it ahead of all other Rubber Bases. It is made of the best Para Gum, which is carefully purified. Owing to the great preponderance of Gum in its composition, it is very light in proportion to bulk. Its marked characteristics are STRENGTH and ELASTICITY, and even at the additional cost it is cheaper than the Red Rubbers, as a much thinner plate is required.

The EXTRA TOUGH RUBBER is susceptible of a very high polish. A sample will be sent free on application, as it is our desire to give ocular proof of its qualities. It vulcanizes in 55 minutes, at 320 degrees Fahrenheit.

THE DENTAL COLLEGE

—OF THE—

UNIVERSITY OF MICHIGAN.

The Eighth Annual Session of this Institution will commence on the 1st of October and close on the last Wednesday of March, thus making a course of six months. The regular course of instructions commence at once, and will proceed through the term, with the customary vacation.

The students in this department will receive instructions in Anatomy, Physiology, Pathology, Chemistry, Materia Medica, Therapeutics, and Surgery, from the Professors of their respective branches in the *Department of Medicine aud Surgery* of the University, when lectures commence, and continue the same as with the Dental College. There will also, in addition, be a special course upon each of these branches. The courses will each embrace from ten to fifteen lectures.

FACULTY OF THE DENTAL DEPARTMENT.

J. B. ANGELL, LL. D.,	President
J. TAFT, M. D., D. D. S.,	Principles and Practice of Operative Dentistry
CORYDON L. FORD, M. D., D. D. S.,	Anatomy and Physiology
J. A. WATLING, D. D. S.,	Clinical and Mechanical Dentistry
W. H. DORRANCE, D. D. S.,	Prosthetic Dentistry
U. D. BILLMEYER, D. D. S.,	Demonstrator of Clinical Dentistry
C. S. CASE, D. D. S.,	Demonstrator of Prosthetic Dentistry

Special instructions will be given in Dental Pathology, Oral Surgery, Dental Therapeutics, and Diseases of women and children with reference to the teeth.

Students should be promptly present at the College on Friday, September 29th, at ten o'clock, A. M., to make the preliminary arrangements for entering upon regular work. Seats in the lecture room are assigned by selection to students in the order of registration on the Steward's books; and each student is expected to occupy, during the session, such seat as he may select. Students, on arriving in Ann Arbor, should call at the Steward's office.

CONDITIONS OF GRADUATION.

The candidate must be twenty-one years of age. *He must furnish satisfactory evidence of good moral character.*

He must devote three years to the study of his profession. He must attend two full courses of Lectures in the Dental College, or one course in some college having an equal standard of requirements, and the last one here, and we recommend that he attend three courses regularly.

He must sustain an examination satisfactory to the Faculty in all the branches taught.

A graduate of the Medical College may enter the Senior Class, and, if found qualified, may graduate after one year has been devoted to the study of Dentistry.

FEES AND EXPENSES.

The Fees, which must be paid in advance, are as follows:

RESIDENTS OF MICHIGAN.—Matriculation Fee, $10 00; annual dues, $25 00.

NON-RESIDENTS.—Matriculation, $25 00; annual dues, $35 00.

GRADUATION FEE.—For all alike, $10 00. The admission fee is paid but once, and entitles the student to the privileges of permanent membership in any department of the University. The annual due is paid the first year and every year thereafter while at the University.

For further particulars, address the Dean of the Dental College, Ann Arbor, Mich.

J. TAFT, Dean.

Codman & Shurtleff's

New

ARTICULATOR

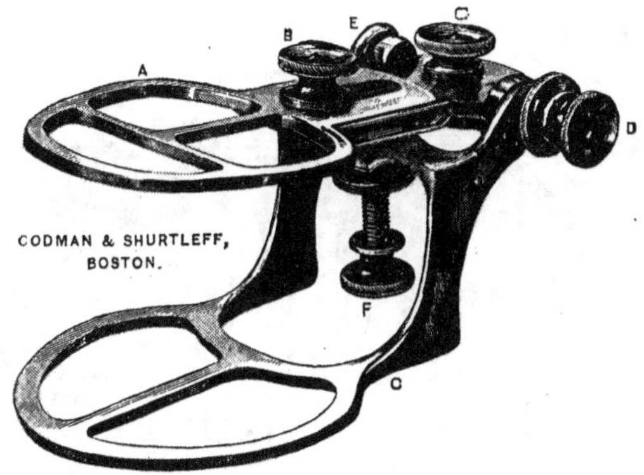

This, we believe, is the latest and best in the market. It is carefully made, and combines many improvements, as will be seen by the description. One special advantage is that each movement can be made entirely independent of every other one.

The upper Jaw A, slides backward and forward in grooves, so that by loosening the Screw B, this motion can be obtained without danger of lateral displacement. There is a second plate upon which the Jaw A moves laterally, and is controlled by the Screw G, so that either of these important motions can be obtained entirely independent of the other. The Screw F, which adjusts the spaces between the Jaws A and C, is provided with a set nut which prevents it from unscrewing. Screws D and E, which form the hinge, are cone pointed, and furnished with set nuts, so that the wear can be taken up, and the movement always kept accurate. On Plate A there is a series of graduating marks by which the dentist can see just how much change. he has made in the articulation.

Price, Plated, - - $2 50.

Codman & Shurtleff's

INHALER

FOR NITROUS OXIDE GAS.

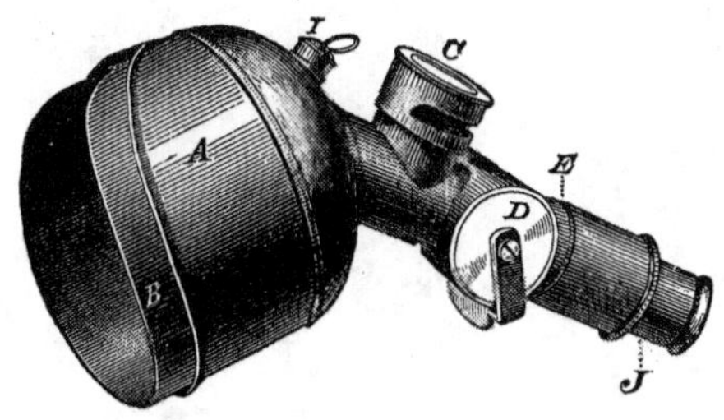

For convenience both to patient and operator, this Inhaler is unequalled. With one hand the dentist can apply the instrument and open or close the stop-cock, leaving the other hand at liberty to control the patient or for such exigencies as may occur.

As the elastic hood covers both nose and mouth, it is not necessary to close the nostrils by clamps or otherwise, thus saving the patient from that feeling of suffocation which is always disagreeable, and to sensitive people positively frightful.

A is the Metal Hood containing B the Flexible Rubber Hood which covers both nose and mouth; C, Exhaling Valve; D, Two-way Stop-cock; I, Packing through which the cord passes that is attached to the Hard Rubber Gag to keep the mouth open. This may be used or not, at the option of the dentist.

A great many of these Inhalers have been sold, and never fail to give satisfaction.

Price Reduced to $10.00.

GIDEON SIBLEY,

Manufacturer of	And Dealer in
ARTIFICIAL TEETH,	**DENTAL SUPPLIES.**

Thirteenth and Filbert Streets, Philadelphia, Pa.

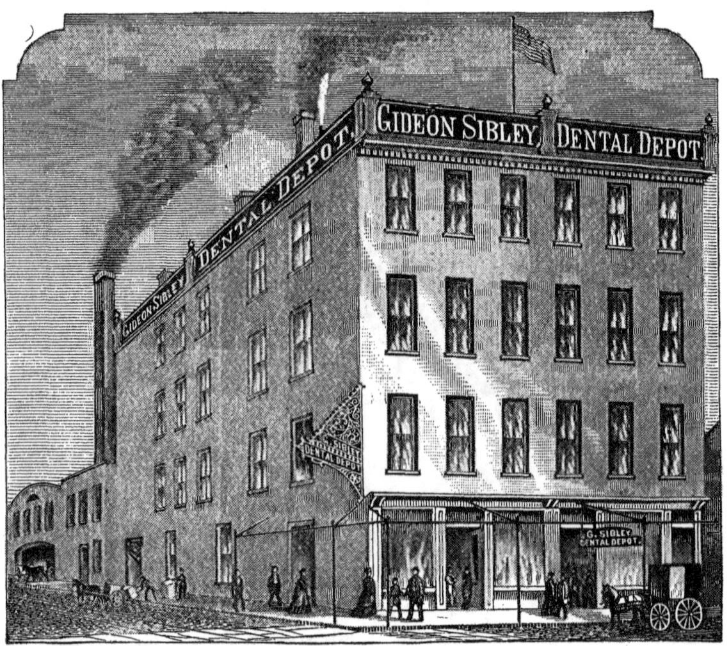

It is gratifying to find, that after years of assiduous labor, to produce the best Tooth made, that their superiority is so universally acknowledged, and that the rapid demand for them has necessitated large additions to our FACTORY and SALES-ROOM.

Points on which We Seek Comparison:

STRENGTH, NATURAL SHAPES, TEXTURE, COLORS, LARGE DOUBLE HEADED PINS, ETC., combined with our very large assortment of MOULDS and variety of SHADES.

☞ Ask your Dealer for them, or send us ONE DOLLAR for a Sample Set.

For Sale by F. S. ACKERMAN & CO., Detroit, Mich.

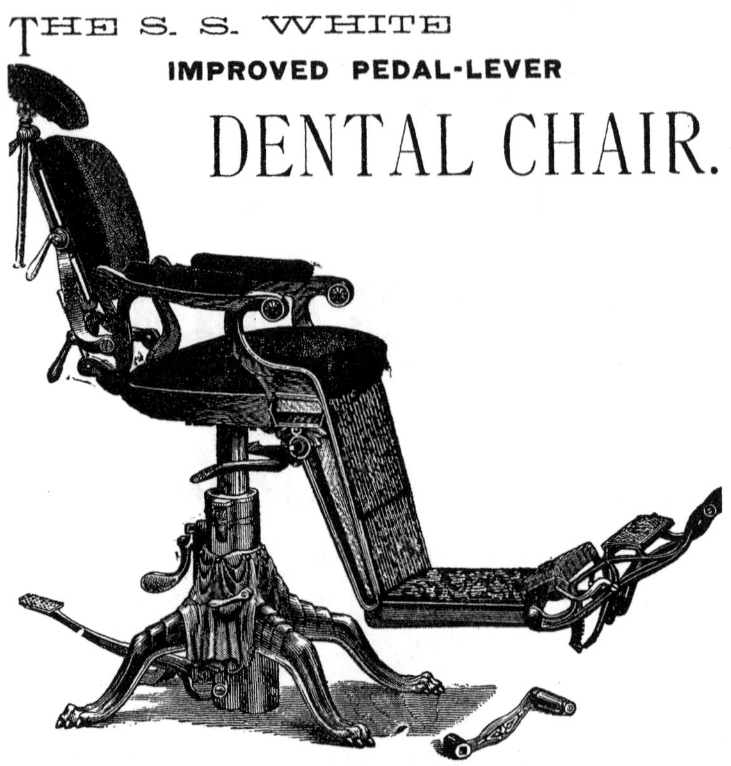

Manufactured under the following Patents: Patented December 28, 1875; October 31, 1876; August 20, 1878; November 26, 1878; November 25, 1879; February 10, 1880; April 12, 1881: April 19, 1881. In England—July 26, 1879. Re-Issues—July 4, 1876; March 19, 1878; June 25, 1878; August 27, 1878.

PRICES:

In best quality Green, Crimson or Maroon Plush	$ 180 00
In either color of finest Plush, puffed with Plush, trimmed with Silk Cord with Wilton Carpet	200 00
In Fancy Upholstering, full Turkish Style, puffed with Plush, and trimmed with Silk Cord, with Carpet to match . . .	210 00
In Crimson Plain Turkey Morocco or Leather	180 00
In Embossed Turkey Morocco, Tan or Crimson, puffed with Plain Morocco, edged with Cord, Axminster Carpet on Apron and Foot-Rests	210 00

BOXING FREE.

Summer Seats of Cane or Perforated Wood	6 00
Extra Backs of Cane	9 00
Linen Covers for Seat, Arms, Back and Head rest	4 00

The cost of freight being at the expense of the buyer, our branch houses and dealers will be obliged to sell at the above prices, with this added.

The S. S. WHITE Dental Manufacturing Co.,
PHILADELPHIA, NEW YORK, BOSTON, CHICAGO, BROOKLYN.

WILKERSON
DENTAL CHAIR.

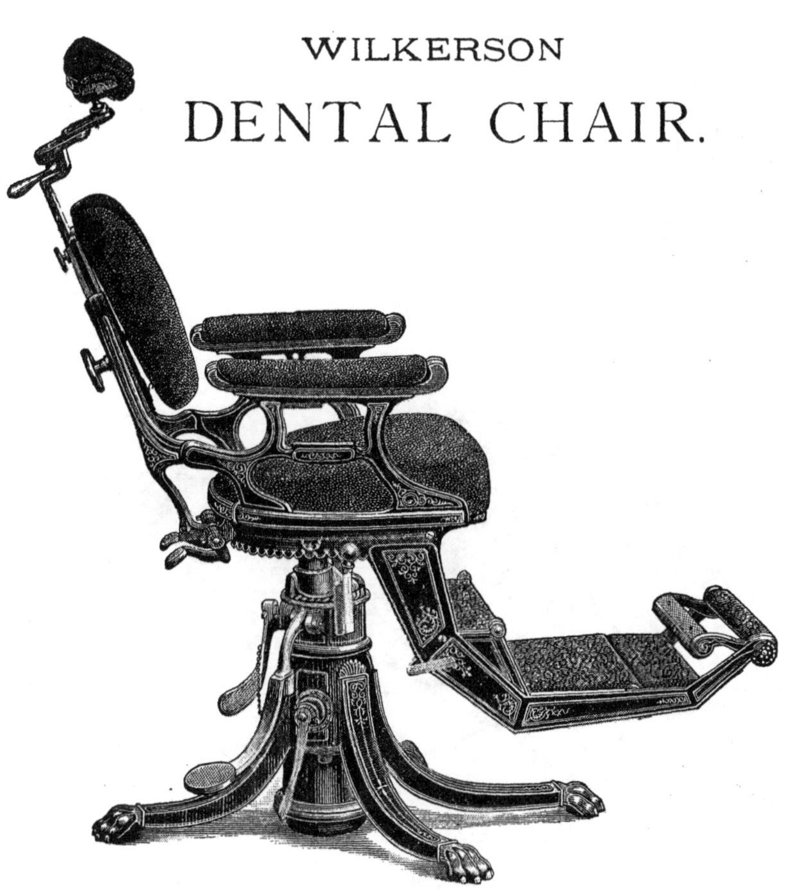

Patented November 20, 1877. Re-Issues—July 4, 1876; October 31, 1876; March 19, 1878; June 25, 1878: August 20, 1878; August 27, 1878.

PRICES:

In best quality Green, Crimson, or Maroon Blush	$ 180 00
In either color of finest Plush, puffed with Plush, trimmed with Silk Cord, with Wilton Carpet	200 00
In Fancy Upholstering, full Turkish Style, puffed with Plush, and trimmed with Silk Cord, with Carpet to match	210 00
In Crimson Plain Turkey Morocco or Leather	180 00
In Embossed Turkey Morocco, Tan or Crimson, puffed with Plain Morocco, edged with Cord, Axminster Carpet on Apron and Foot-Rests	210 00

BOXING FREE.

The cost of freight being at the expense of the buyer, our branch houses and dealers will be obliged to sell at the above prices, with this added.

The S. S. WHITE Dental Manufacturing Co.,
PHILADELPHIA, NEW YORK, BOSTON, CHICAGO, BROOKLYN.

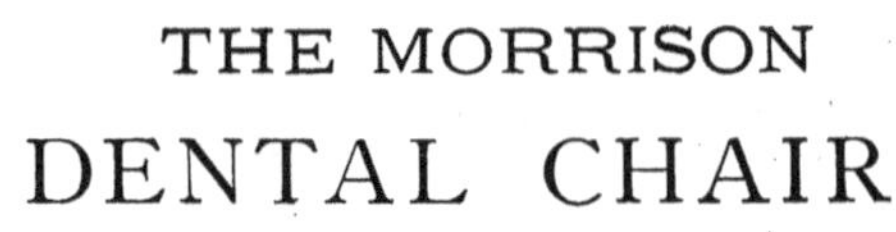

THE MORRISON DENTAL CHAIR.

Re-Issue May 15. 1877.
English Patent, Dec. 7, 1867.

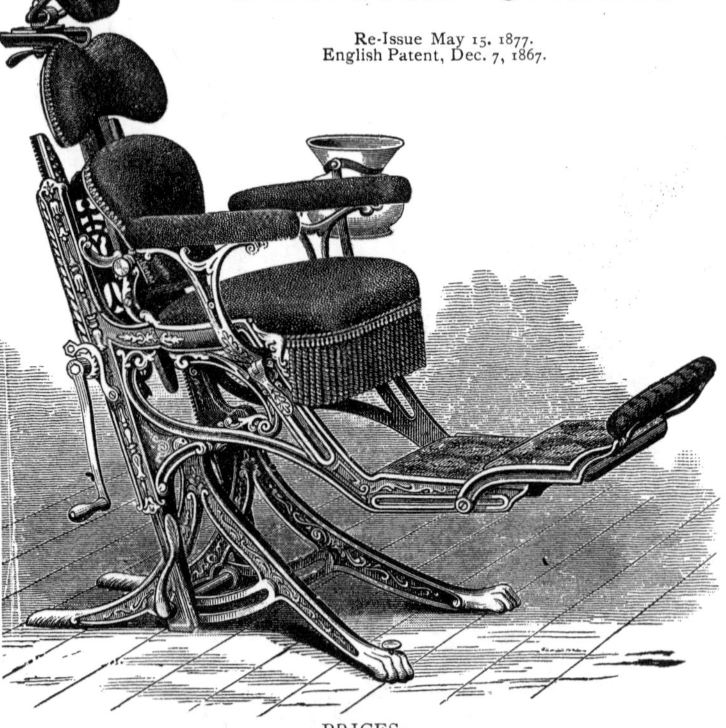

PRICES:

In best quality Green or Garnet Plush	$ 130 00
In Real Morocco, Embossed	140 00
In finest quality Green or Garnet Plush, pufled and trimmed with Silk Plush, full Turkish Upholstery	150 00
In French Moquet, Bouquet pattern	145 00
In same, but puffed with Silk Plush, full Turkish Upholstery . .	160 00

BOXING FREE:

STUDENT'S MORRISON CHAIR.

To meet an often-expressed want of a first-class chair at a low price, the Student's Morrison was brought out. It is, in all respects, equal to the regular Morrison chair, except that it is upholstered in a seal-brown corded material, instead of a plush. It presents a very neat appearance, and will wear nearly as well as plush.

PRICE:

In Corded Upholstery . . . . $ 105 00

We supply either style of the Morrison Chair, with or without Casters. When ordered with Casters, the price is $10 00 extra.

The S. S. WHITE Dental Manufacturing Co.,
PHILADELPHIA, NEW YORK, BOSTON, CHICAGO, BROOKLYN.

SURGEON'S CASE,

Nos. 1 and 2.

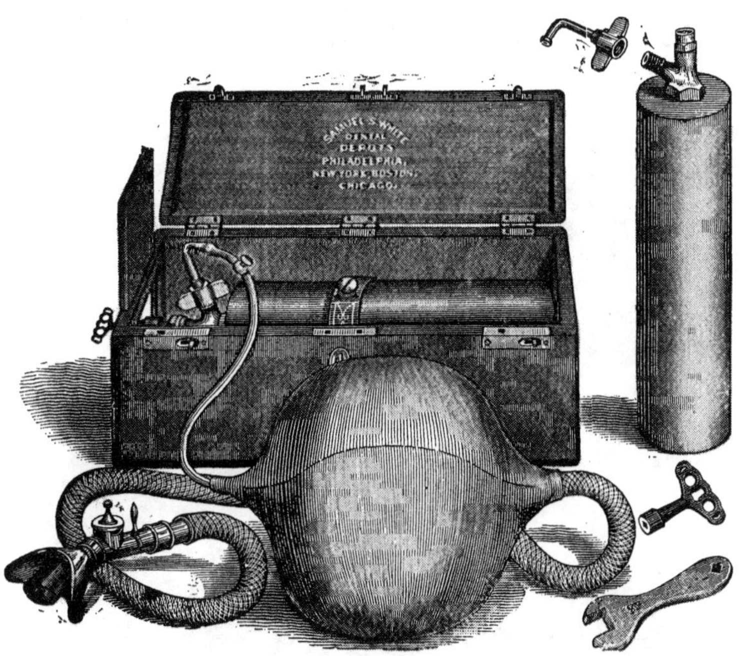

The complete apparatus is shown in cut, and consists of an iron cylinder containing at least 100 gallons, (usually more) of nitrous oxide, liquefied, to which is attached the necessary tubing, gas-bag, and inhaler; the whole inclosed in a stout morocco case lined with velvet.

In manufacturing the Surgeon's Case particular attention has been given to each and every part, so as to insure not only a complete but the very best apparatus of its kind.

The Case is made of well-seasoned wood, is lined with velvet, and covered with morocco, and the hinges lock, and bolts are nickle-plated. A stout cast-steel ring, neatly japanned, with a heavy set-screw, clamps the cylinder.

The No. 1 Case has a 4½-gallon bag, and the No. 2 case has a 7-gallon bag.

PRICES:

No. 1 Case, complete, with Filled Cylinder . . . . . . $ 42 00
" 2 " " " " " 44 00

The S. S. WHITE Dental Manufacturing Co.,
PHILADELPHIA, NEW YORK, BOSTON, CHICAGO, BROOKLYN.

UPRIGHT
SURGEON'S CASE,

Nos. 3, 4, 5 and 6.

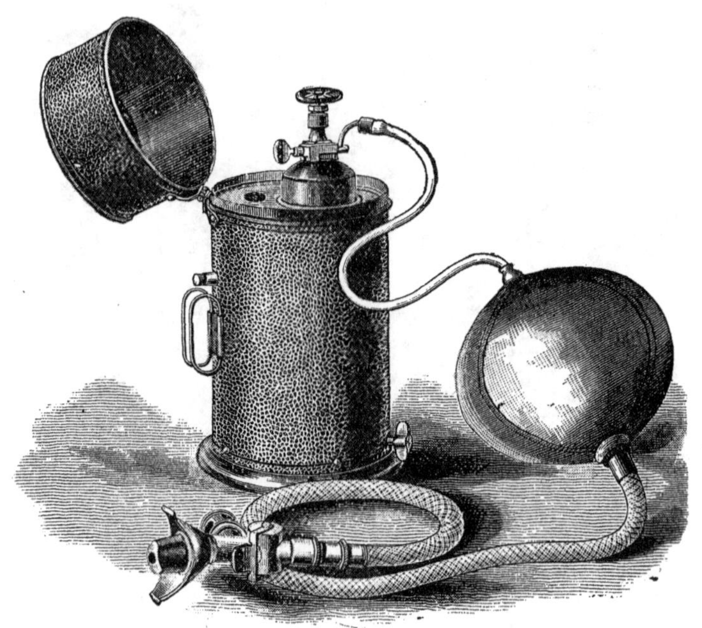

In this form of Case the cylinder stands on end, which is reckoned by some operators an advantage in permitting a free flow of gas, but we have had no complaints of the original form as shown in Cases Nos. 1 and 2. To meet all demands we offer the two forms.

No. 3, Complete Apparatus, with 4½-gallon bag in stout Tin Case, covered with Leather	$ 42 00
No. 4, the same, but with 7-gallon bag	44 00
No. 5, Complete Apparatus, with 4½-gallon Bag in stout Tin Case, handsomely Japanned	36 00
No. 6, the same, but with 7-gallon bag	38 00

TRIPOD. STAND.

Invention of W. H. Downs.

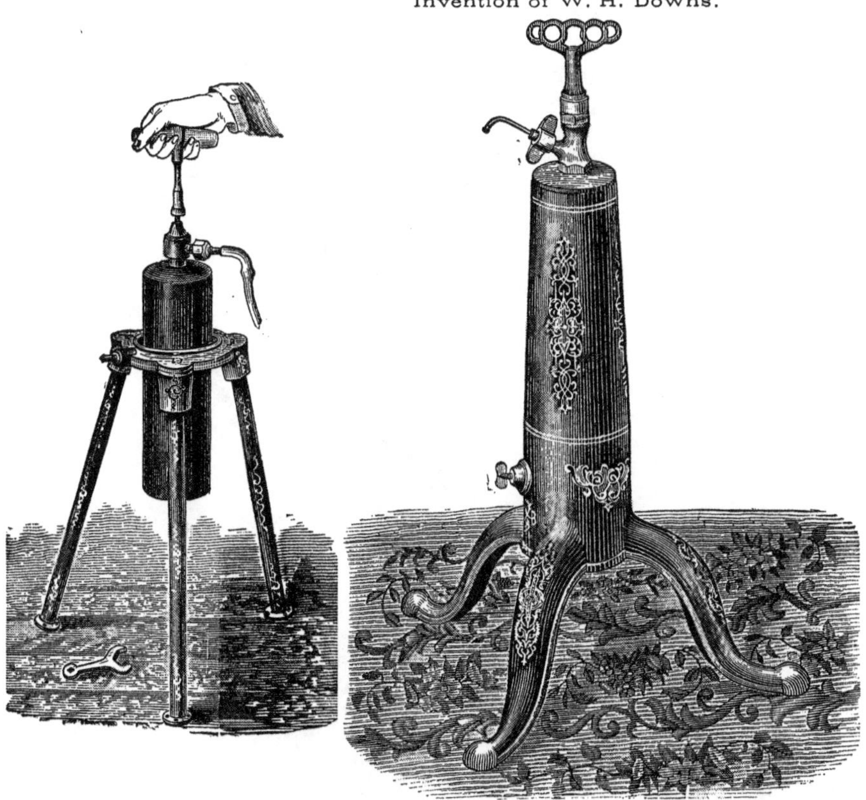

These are simple and convenient devices for holding gas cylinders, and are specially designed for use in the operating room of the resident dentist.

The Tripod consists of an iron ring into which are screwed three pieces of iron pipe.

The Stand consists of an iron base with a tin casing in which the cylinder is placed and securely held by a set-screw.

Both Tripod and Stand are japanned and ornamented.

PRICES:

Tripod for 100-gallon Cylinder	$ 4 00
Stand " 100- " "	7 00
" " 500- " "	9 00
Tripod with 100- " " (filled), Bag, Tubing and Inhaler .	34 00
Stand " 100- " " " " " " " .	37 00
" " 500- " " " " " " " .	68 00

The prices of 500-gallon Cylinders may vary slightly, as the Gas, whether more or less than 500 Gallons, is charged at 4½ cents per gallon.

The S. S. WHITE Dental Manufacturing Co.,
PHILADELPHIA, NEW YORK, BOSTON, CHICAGO, BROOKLYN.

FOIL CLIPPER.

PATENTED FEBRUARY 1, 1881.

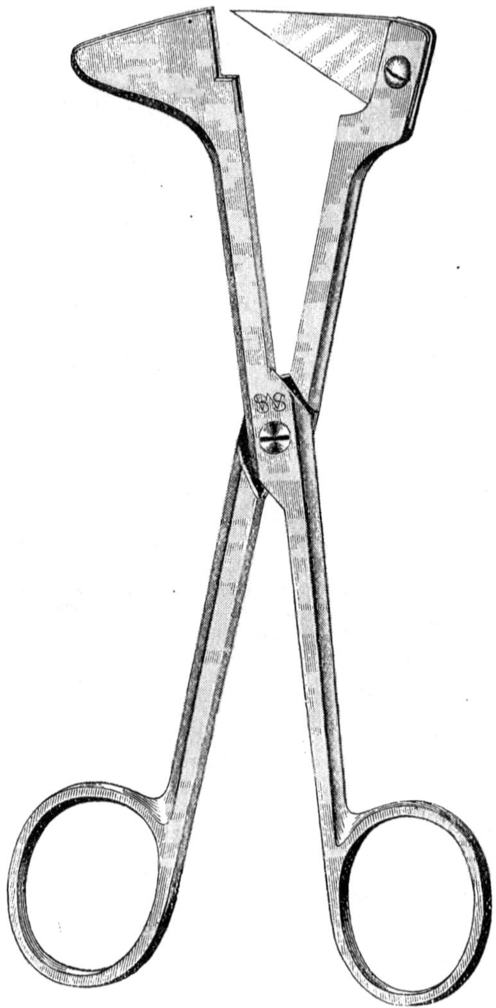

This Clipper is designed for cutting ropes of gold foil into small pieces or cylinders, and is the only cutting-instrument on sale which will successfully cut foil without condensing it. Shears and scissors, however sharp they may be ground, will condense and harden the gold, but by the use of this Clipper, the edges are left soft and free.

Price, Nickel-plated . . . . $ 2 00

The S. S. WHITE Dental Manufacturing Co.,
PHILADELPHIA, NEW YORK, BOSTON, CHICAGO, BROOKLYN.

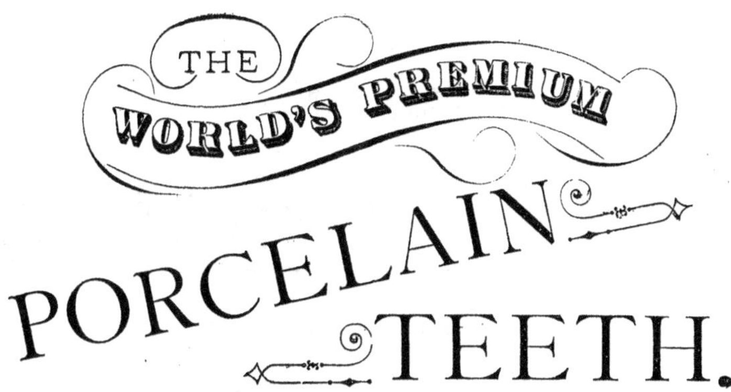

THIRTY-SEVEN years ago SAMUEL S. WHITE'S PORCELAIN TEETH were recognized as the best that had been made up to that time. From then until now they have steadily maintained the leading position, their superiority over all others being attested by the receipt of the ***highest award at each of the Great World's Fairs, from the first, held in London in 1851, to the latest, recently closed in Melbourne.*** Other manufacturers have *claimed* the same distinction, but a reference to the lists of awards will satisfy any one that wherever graded premiums have been given, we have uniformly received the highest in our class. Thus, at Vienna, the highest award was the

GRAND DIPLOMA OF HONOR.

We received the *only* one given to a manufacturer of Porcelain Teeth. Again, at Paris, in 1878, the highest prize was the Gold Medal. We received the *only* one in our class.

We claim, and the facts sustain the claim, that our teeth, in the varied points of excellence which go to make up the perfect substitute for the natural organs—texture, translucency, individual and relative form, with reference to imitation of nature's types—are decidedly and unmistakably superior to any others.

In forms, sizes, and shades, our stock presents an unapproached variety. Natures variations are as numerous as are individuals. We do not pretend to rival nature, but no other manufacturer offers equal opportunities for selection of teeth to meet differences in age, complexion, physical conformation, and other peculiarities of individual cases, whether for metal, rubber, celluloid, or porcelain base.

In gum sections we have, besides an immense stock of the ordinary types, many new and desirable combinations for full and partial dentures. Of those for partial cases we may name, centrals in pairs, a central and a lateral (right or left) in pairs, two centrals and a lateral (right or left), bicuspids in pairs, etc.

Our assortment of plain teeth for celluloid work is very fine.

We have also the approved forms, new and old, of porcelain crowns for attachment to natural roots, including the Bonwill & Gates, the Weston, the Richmond and the Foster crowns.

Porcelain cavity-stoppers are a late development wherewith lost portions of crowns may be replaced simply and effectively with porcelain.

The S. S. WHITE Dental Manufacturing Co.,
PHILADELPHIA, NEW YORK, BOSTON, CHICAGO, BROOKLYN

ROBINSON'S

FIBROUS AND TEXTILE

METALLIC FILLING

For the Teeth and for Lining

Robinson's Improved

PATENT DENTAL PLATE.

A NEW MATERIAL.

For Sale by F. S. ACKERMAN & CO.

The thoughtful and observing dentists have long been aware of the injurious and in many cases fatal effects of wearing rubber plates for artificial teeth, and yet it is the common material used in this country and in Europe for artificial dentures. The ease and convenience with which rubber work has been made, and the general apparent utility, has brought it into use for the millions in all countries.

There have been very few rubber workers, and a less number of persons who wear rubber plates that have known that the make-up of rubber for vulcanite purposes is composed of 40% rubber, 24% sulphur, and 36% mercury, and that the combination is *sulphuret of mercury.* It is natural that such a combination should produce injurious effects upon peculiar and susceptible constitutions. Now whether the sulphuret of mercury or the heat generated by wearing a vegetable plate produces the effect described or not, the fact remains that in all cases where rubber is worn, the mucus surface becomes inflamed, and in many cases it is unbearable, and in all cases positively injurious. Some two years ago Dr. Robinson, of Jackson, became so impressed with the importance of something necessary to remedy this evil, that after much experimenting, he succeeded in making a metal lining for rubber and celluloid plates for which he has obtained a patent. These new metallic lined plates not only cure all inflamed mouths in a very short time, and take away all that heat and tired feeling so often experienced by persons wearing rubber who are nervous and delicate, but make a plate as good and perfect as gold or platinum, with very little additional expense to those who are obliged to wear artificial sets of teeth. This same material discovered for the lining of the plates, is the best material known for filling teeth, if we except gold, and in many cases, in combination with gold, better than gold itself, on account of its extreme ductility and adaptation to the walls of the tooth.

In offering this material to the dentists, and the public, the proprietor claims that it is, in the following particulars, superior to anything ever yet brought before the profession, and will supply a need long felt by every careful and experienced dentist:

1. The material is so soft that it is more easily introduced into difficult places between the teeth than *any other metallic filling*.

2. There is absolutely no recoil when placed in a cavity under hand pressure or the mallet.

3. It is more certain of seccessful results in the hands of persons who cannot make first-class operations with gold.

4. It does not soil or change color in the mouth.

5. The welding properties are greater than any preparation except sponge gold.

6. Gold welds to it as readily as gold welds to itself.

7. It finishes easier than gold, and retains a fine and brilliant polish.

8. It is superior for buccal, lingual and cervical walls, and in conjunction, or interlocked with gold, will make a better filling than gold itself.

9. It is a saving of more than half the expense and time.

10. This material, though fibrous like Felt Foil, *is not* Felt Foil, as it contains no mercury.

11. It is less of a conductor than gold, and there is less danger of trouble from thermal changes in large cavities with the walls lightly covering the nerves.

12. In working this material, coarse and sharp serrated points should be used, as everyone is aware that where the serrates are deep there is more surface of the metal to come in contact; and all pure metals will unite by heat and pressure when the surfaces are free from oxidation.

DIAMOND STATE TOOTH MANUFACTORY.

THE WILMINGTON

Dental Manufacturing Co.,

MANUFACTURERS OF SUPERIOR

ARTIFICIAL TEETH.

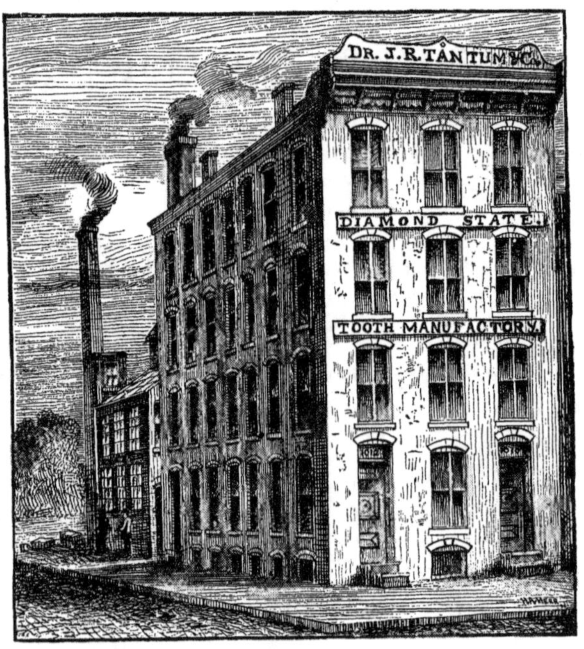

Office and Factory, 1010 & 1012 King Street, WILMINGTON, DELAWARE.

BRANCH DEPOT:

340 Fulton Street, Brooklyn, New York.

TRUE MERIT our claim. We ask for our teeth a trial at your hands, an HONEST TEST, and then we fear not the verdict. Ask your nearest dealer for them or send ONE DOLLAR for trial set to

THE WILMINGTON DENTAL MANUFACTURING CO.,

909 Market Street, Wilmington, Delaware.

For Sale by F. S. ACKERMAN & CO., Michigan Dental Depot.

SAMSON RUBBER

MANUFACTURED BY

EUGENE DOHERTY,

444 First Street, BROOKLYN, E. D., New York.

WARRANTED TO BE

THE STRONGEST AND MOST UNIFORM RUBBER MANUFACTURED.

It is the TOUGHEST and Most Durable Rubber Made.
Vulcanizes same as Ordinary Rubber.

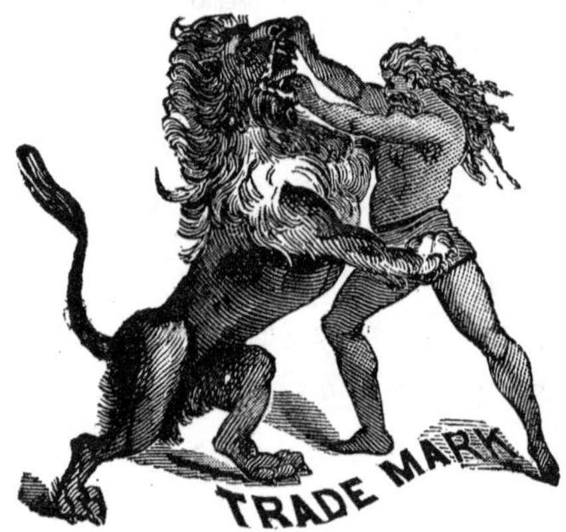

MANUFACTURER OF ALL KINDS OF

DENTAL RUBBERS AND GUTTA PERCHAS

PRICE LIST OF DENTAL RUBBERS AND GUTTA PERCHAS.

No. 1 Rubber, per lb. -	$2 50	No. 1 Weighted or Amalgamated Rubber, per lb. - -	$4 00
No. 2 Rubber, per lb. - -	2 50	No. 2 Weighted or Amalgamated Rubber, per lb. - -	4 00
Samson Rubber, per lb. -	3 00	Black Weighted or Amalgamated Rubber, per lb. - -	4 00
Black Rubber, per lb. - -	2 50	Weighted Gutta Percha, per lb.	4 00
Flexible or Palate Rubber, per lb.	2 75	Adamantine Filling or Stopping.	
Gutta Percha for Bass Plates, per lb. - - - - -	2 50		
Vulcanite Gutta Percha, per lb.	3 50		

NOTE.—The above Rubbers and Gutta Perchas will be furnished in pound or half-pound packages to any Dentist in the country on receipt of price, and stating that they cannot get them at the Dental Depot in or near their place of business. Circulars giving full instructions how to use all my Rubbers and Gutta Perchas, will be found in each package of the article ordered.

EUGENE DOHERTY,
444 First St., Brooklyn, E. D., New York.

For Sale by F. S. ACKERMAN & CO., Detroit, Mich.

H. D. JUSTI'S

IMPROVED HAND SOCKET HOLDERS AND HANDLES.

Patented February 18th, 1868.
" April 29th, 1879.

Re-issued July 8th, 1879.

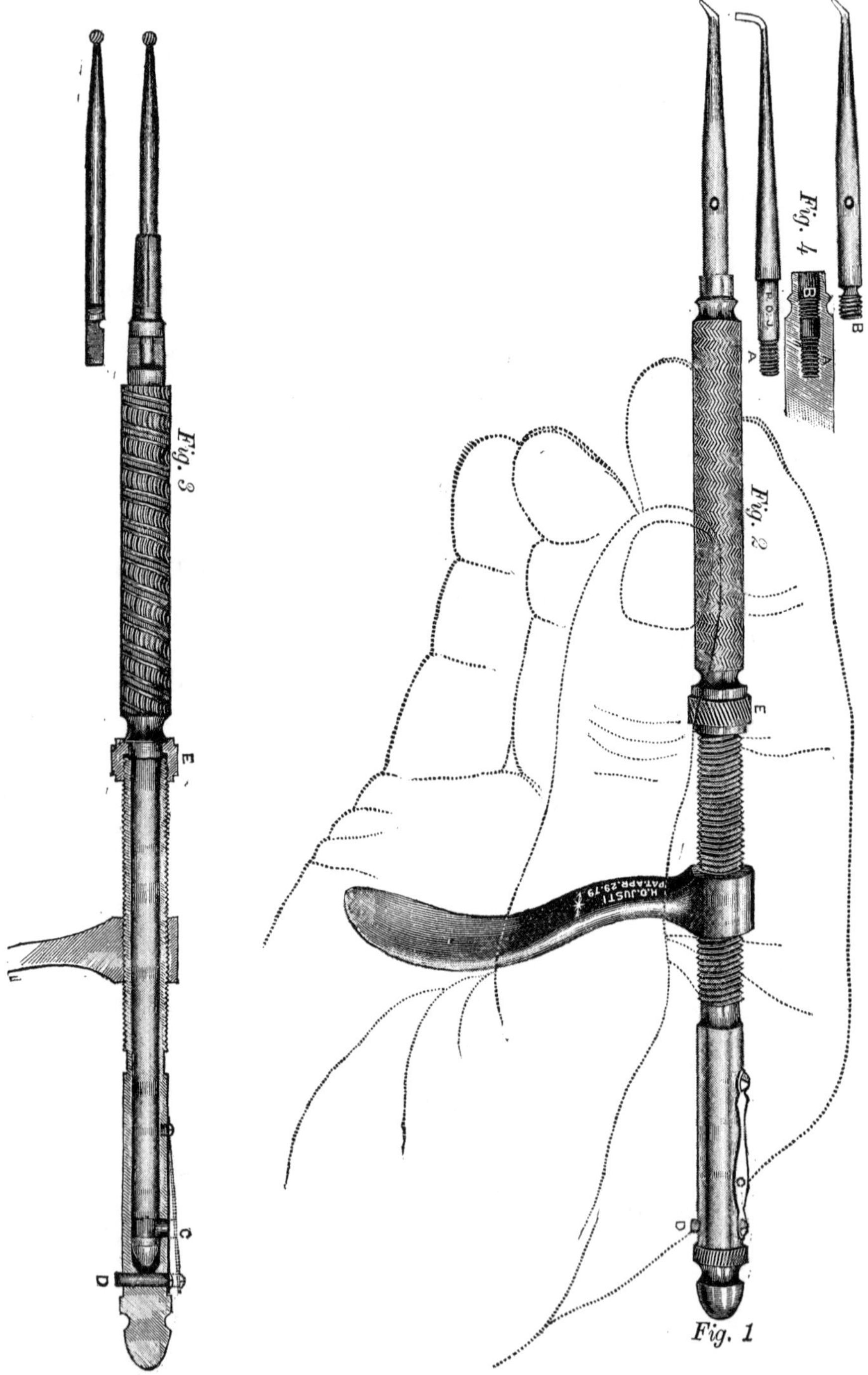

H. D. JUSTI'S
IMPROVED HAND SOCKET HOLDERS AND HANDLES.

Patented February 18th, 1868. Re-issued July 8th, 1879.
" April 29th, 1879.

Fig. 1 & 2 shows the holder and handle complete, adapted to receive Plugger and Excavator Points. Fig. 3 shows sectional view of holder with handle to receive Engine Points. Fig. 4 shows part section of handle threaded to correspond with thread on points A & B.

Note.—The points should invariably be fastened in the handles with pliers designed for that purpose, to make them firm and prevent slipping.

These Instruments were introduced by me several years ago with a fixed socket handle, adapted to receive Pluggers, Excavators and Engine Points. The general satisfaction, which they gave to the Profession over the old Hand pressure Instruments, through their ease and facility of manipulation, attested to by their numerous and increased sales and testimonials, has induced me to make several valuable improvements in the same, adapting them to receive not only Excavators, Plugger Points, &c. of my own manufacture, but also the Snow & Lewis, and other Points in general use, by which those who have been using other Socket Instruments, and wish to substitute my improved ones, may still make use of their old points.

The handles instead of being fixed to the Socket holder, (necessitating the changing of points for the various positions of cavities, as formerly), may now be changed instantly, (by means of the small spring C, Fig. 3), with the desired point already screwed in. By this method the point can be screwed in firmly, and need only be removed if it requires repairing.

The holder has also been furnished with a small jam-nut, (E, Fig. 1 & 3); take the holder in the right hand, at its extreme end, and give the nut several turns to the right, this will effectually prevent the Instrument from rotating, which is very important where great solidity of gold is desired, as it makes the Instrument firmer, thus preventing possible slipping.

The Instrument consists of a Socket holder, (see Fig. 1), in which the handles (Fig. 2 & 3) are inserted, and where they are retained by the spring C. The holder is provided with a lateral arm adapted to fit in the palm of the hand, and may be lengthened or shortened to adapt it to different size hands.

This arm will enable the operator to apply the entire pressure required, by the body of his hand, instead of the fingers, as formerly, leaving the fingers free to guide and direct the tool.

With all other Instruments made, the entire strain and pressure is received by the ends of the fingers, which soon become cramped and tired.

For plugging and drilling, the Socket holder is invaluable, and is also very desirable for excavating and chiseling, the arm acting as a support, thereby enabling you to use more force when cutting, without fear of slipping and thus lascerating the gum.

I have constantly on hand a large variety of points to fit these handles, such as Pluggers, Excavators and Engine Points, which may be ordered from any catalogue or price list, and will be furnished at manufacturers prices.

DIRECTIONS.

The Instrument is grasped in the usual manner, with the point between the thumb and fingers, whereupon the body of the Socket holder will rest across the outside of the hand, and the arm leans against the palm, in which position the Instrument is ready for use; the fingers being used to guide the point, and the body of the hand to give the pressure. The lateral arm can be raised or lowered to suit the size of the hand, as shown in Fig. 1. To change the handle, take the holder in one hand, pressing on the end D, of the small latch spring C, with pivot attached, which thus releases handle.

Branch,

66 MADISON STREET, CHICAGO, ILL.

H. D. JUSTI,

DENTAL DEPOT,

516 Arch Street, Philadelph'

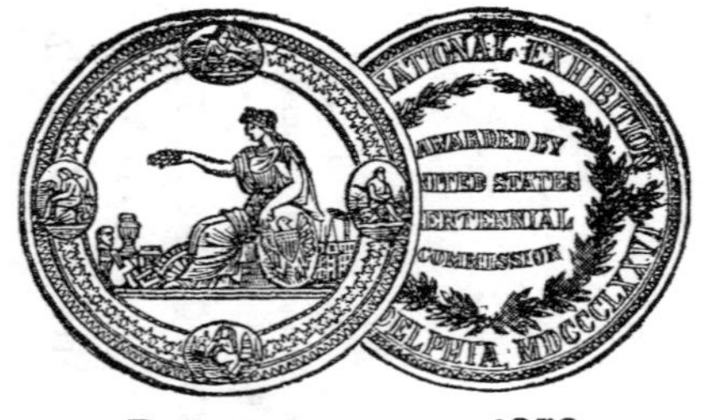

PHILADELPHIA, 1876.

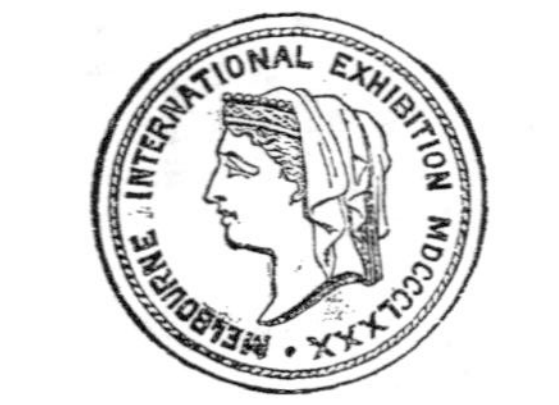

MELBOURNE, 1880.

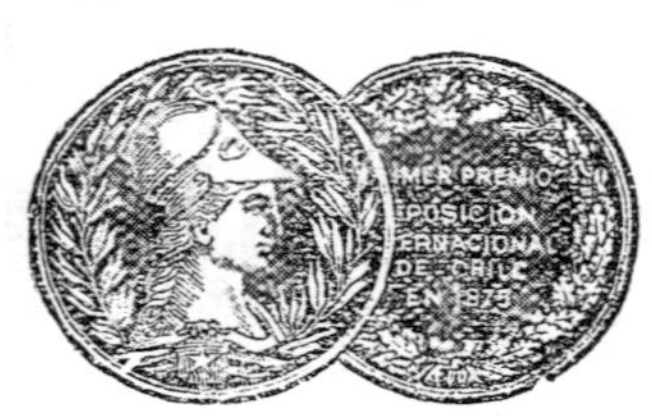

SANTIAGO DE CHILI, 1875.

SYDNEY

INTERNATIONAL EXHIBITION

1879

CERTIFICATE OF AWARD

ARTIFICIAL TEETH

H. D. JUSTI.

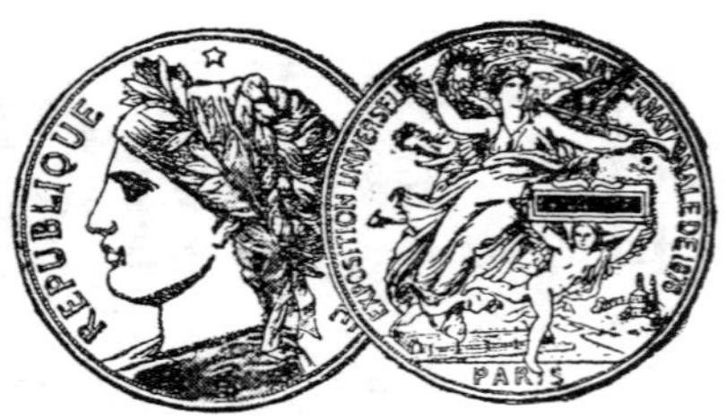

PARIS, 1878.

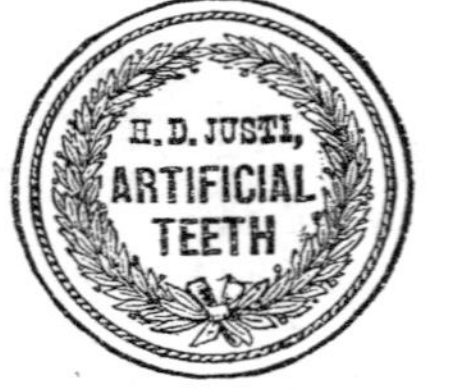

MELBOURNE, 1880.

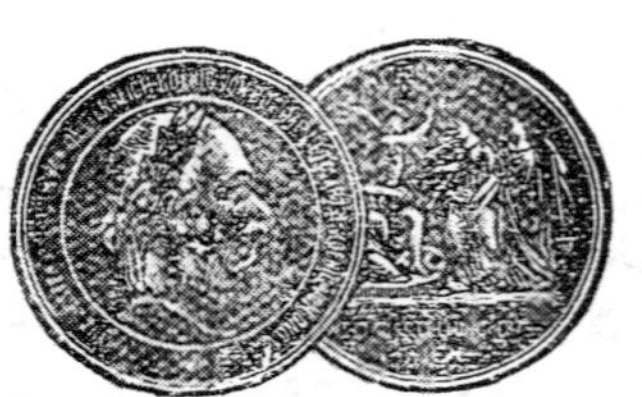

VIENNA, 1873.

www.ingramcontent.com/pod-product-compliance
Lightning Source LLC
LaVergne TN
LVHW011203110826
845150LV00006B/1304

* 9 7 8 1 4 2 5 5 1 8 5 8 5 *